OCCUPATIONAL AND ENVIRONMENTAL MEDICINE
SELF-ASSESSMENT REVIEW

OCCUPATIONAL AND ENVIRONMENTAL MEDICINE
SELF-ASSESSMENT REVIEW

Robert J. McCunney, M.D.
Director, Environmental Medical Service
Massachusetts Institute of Technology
Cambridge, Massachusetts

Paul P. Rountree, M.D.
Associate Professor
Occupational and Environmental Medicine
Occupational Health Sciences
University of Texas Health Center at Tyler
Tyler, Texas

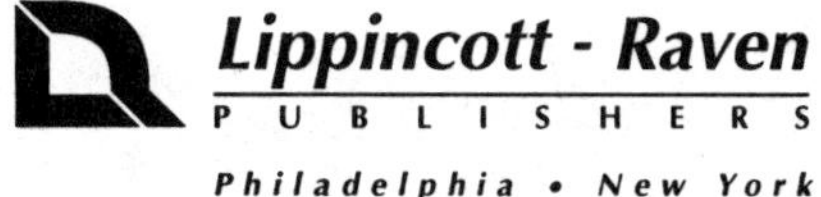

Lippincott - Raven
PUBLISHERS
Philadelphia • New York

Acquisitions Editor: Joyce-Rachel John
Developmental Editor: Delois Patterson
Manufacturing Manager: Kevin Watt
Production Manager: Robert Pancotti
Production Editor: Jeff Somers
Indexer: Prottsman Indexing
Compositor: Lippincott–Raven Desktop Division
Printer: Victor Graphics

Printed in the United States of America

9 8 7 6 5 4 3 2 1

Library of Congress Cataloging-in-Publication Data
McCunney, Robert J.
    Occupational and environmental medicine : self-assessment review /
Robert J. McCunney, Paul P. Rountree.
      p.   cm.
    Includes bibliographical references and index.
    ISBN 0-7817-1612-8 (alk. paper)
    1. Medicine.   Industrial--Examinations, questions, etc. 2. Environmental health--Examinations, questions, etc.
    I.   Rountree, Paul P. II.   Title.
    [DNLM: 1.   Occupational Medicine examination questions.
  2.   Environmental Medicine examination questions.   WA 18.2 M478o
1998]
RC963.3.M23 1998
616.9′803′076--dc21
DNLM/DLC
for Library of Congress   98-5990
                                           CIP

Contents

Preface

Our patients frequently question us about perceived relationships between disease and exposures from their work or environment. They ask, will my job cause me to get cancer? Why can't my wife get pregnant? Did fumes or dust from my workplace cause my lung condition? These questions, and hundreds like them, are difficult to answer with certainty.

Few doctors are comfortable with issues concerning environmental or workplace hazards. Small wonder! Only about 40% of our medical schools integrate any material about occupational and environmental medicine into their curriculum. Even in those institutions which do, the amount of time devoted over 4 years averages only 4 hours!

In 1966, the prestigious Institute of Medicine recommended additional training in these areas for all primary care physicians. Unfortunately, busy clinicians had only a minimal amount of material available for independent continuing medical education (CME) activity. Two years ago, the American College of Occupational and Enviromental Medicine (ACOEM) encouraged the development of a self assessment program which would allow physicians to earn needed CME credits while engaged in such study.

This book borrows largely from the content of the familiar and popular textbook *A Practical Approach to Occupational and Environmental Medicine (Second Edition)*. A series of questions have been developed from material in that text, and these have been peer-reviewed by an independent panel of ACOEM members.

This book should be of value to primary care physicians, to practicing occupational physicians who would like to assess the current state of their knowledge of the specialty while gaining valuable CME credits in the process, and to those preparing for the board examination in Preventive Medicine-Occupational.

The book required first-rate efforts from a number of people, including Edward J. Bernacki, John P. Gibbs, Jeffrey S. Harris, John D. Meyer, and Mark J. Upfal who served as peer reviewers. Paul P. Roundtree, my friend and colleague, deserves praise for his energy, vision, and persistence. Paul took on this task with vigor and managed to encourage his colleagues to contribute to a text that underwent numerous reviews and revisions prior to completion. It is our hope that this publication will aid physicians in providing high-quality occupational and environmental medical care.

Robert J. McCunney, M.D.

Section Editors

(CHAPTERS 1-10)
Jeffrey L. Levin, M.D., M.S.P.H. *Chairman and Professor, Occupational and Environmental Medicine, Occupational Health Sciences, University of Texas Health Center at Tyler, Tyler, Texas 75710-2003*

(CHAPTERS 11-20)
Jack E. Farnham, M.D., M.P.H. *Associate Professor, Occupational and Environmental Medicine, University of Texas Health Center at Tyler, Tyler, Texas 75710-2003*

(CHAPTERS 21-30)
J. Steven Moore, M.D., M.P.H. *Associate Professor, Occupational and Environmental Medicine, Occupational Health Sciences, University of Texas Health Center at Tyler, Tyler, Texas 75710-2003*

(CHAPTERS 31-40)
Eugenia C. George, M.D. *Associate Professor, Occupational and Environmental Medicine, University of Texas Health Center at Tyler, Tyler, Texas 75710-2003*

(CHAPTERS 41-50)
Arthur L. Frank, M.D., Ph.D. *Associate Director of Medical Education, Topperman Professor of Medical Education, Professor of Occupational and Environmental Medicine, Professor of Cell Biology and Environmental Sciences, University of Texas Health Center at Tyler, Tyler, Texas 75710-2003*

User Instructions for CME Credit

Congratulations on your purchase of the *Occupational and Environmental Medicine: Self-Assessment Review* by Robert J. McCunney and Paul P. Rountree which is designed to be used with *A Practical Approach to Occupational and Environmental Medicine, Second Edition.* Please check your book to ensure that all of the following program materials have been included in your copy of *Occupational and Environmental Medicine: Self-Assessment Review*:

- Answer sheets for Units 1,2,3,4,5
- An evaluation form
- CME request forms

TWO WAYS TO USE THE PROGRAM

1. *Beginning to End...* You can read *A Practical Approach to Occupational and Environmental Medicine, Second Edition,* from cover to cover and complete all the test questions from *Occupational and Environmental Medicine: Self-Assessment Review,* at one time for the entire 75 CMEs.
2. *Review...* You can concentrate on the chapters in *A Practical Approach to Occupational and Environmental Medicine, Second Edition,* that are most relevant to your practice and return the answer sheets for the units completed in *Occupational and Environmental Medicine: Self-Assessment Review* for 15 CMEs per unit.

LEARNING OBJECTIVES

After completing this entire review, the user will understand the following as it relates to occupational medicine:

- scope of practice
- legal and ethical issues
- role of regulatory agencics
- development of worksite occupational health programs and centers
- clinical assessments

- accreditation for health centers
- diseases and disorders common in the workforce
- toxicology
- epidemiology and surveillance
- ergonomics
- environmental health

PROGRAM INFORMATION

- Target Audience: Persons preparing for Boards; Persons desiring to update and check their knowledge base.
- Estimated Time to Complete this CME Program: 75 hours
- Method of Physician Participation: Reading *A Practical Approach to Occupational and Environmental Medicine, Second Edition,* and answering questions found in *Occupational and Environmental Medicine: Self-Assessment Review.*
- Evaluation Methods: Participants will complete and return self-assessment examination forms.

REQUESTS FOR CME

The American College of Occupational and Environmental Medicine (ACOEM) is accredited by the Accreditation Council on Continuing Medical Education to offer continuing medical education credit for educational activity. ACOEM designates each of the five sections of the *Occupational and Environmental Medicine: Self-Assessment Review,* the companion volume to *A Practical Approach to Occupational and Environmental Medicine,* for a maximum of 15 credits in Category 1 of the American Medical Association s Physician s Recognition Award. Thus, completion of the entire self-assessment program may be worth up to 75 CMEs.

Continuing medical education credit can be earned on a one-time-only basis for each section of the *Occupational and Environmental Medicine: Self-Assessment Review.* Physicians may complete sections one at a time. Completion of all five sections or completion of the sections in a particular order is not required to earn CMEs.

The CME credit for each section requires the following:

1. Completion of reading all ten chapters of the relevant section in *A Practical Approach to Occupational and Environmental Medicine.*
2. Completion of reading the objectives, the outlines, and the key points related to each of the chapters of the relevant section of the *Occupational and Environmental Medicine: Self-Assessment Review.*
3. Completion of all questions related to each chapter in *Occupational and Environmental Medicine: Self-Assessment Review.*
4. Self-scoring of all questions cited above with the scores reported.
5. Review of the answer explanations. It is suggested that the answers to all questions are read in entirety to maximize learning and that the references are reread.
6. Completion of the appropriate *Occupational and Environmental Medicine: Self-Assessment Review.* Please note that one form must be completed per unit of the *Review.*

7. The mailing of that form (those forms) and the answer sheet(s) plus a check in the amount of $75 **for each section** or $375 for all five sections *in Occupational and Environmental Medicine: Self Assessment Review* to the following address:

> Department of Education
> CME Coordinator
> The American College of Occupational and Environmental Medicine
> 55 West Seegers Road
> Arlington Heights, IL 60005-3919

Your letter awarding your CME credits should arrive within four (4) weeks.

For questions or concerns, contact the Education Department.

Date of Original Release: July, 1998

Date Credit Expires for this Program, July, 2001

The following CME activity was planned and produced in accordance with the Accreditation Council for Continuing Medical Education's (ACCME) *Standards for Interpreting the Essentials as Applied to Continuing Medical Education Enduring Materials.*

The American College of Occupational and Environmental Medicine certifies that this Continuing Medical Education offering meets the criteria for up to 75 credit hours in Category 1 of the Physician's Recognition Award of the American Medical Association. Each physician should claim only those hours of credit that he/she actually spent in the educational activity.

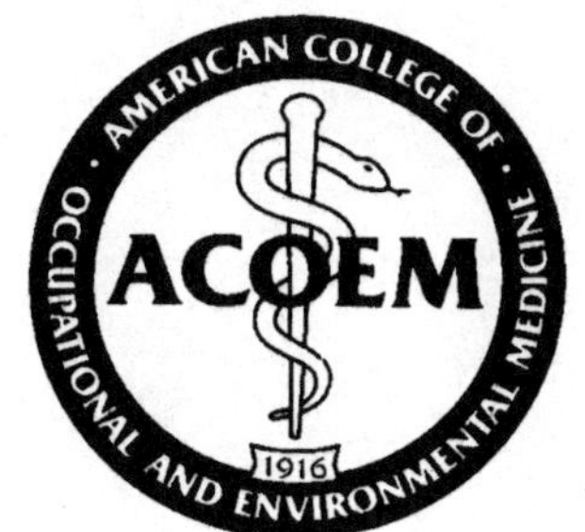

CME Registration for Unit 1 of
Occupational and Environmental Medicine: Self-Assessment Review
Please print clearly.

Name ______________________________________ Medical Degree ______

Address ____________________ City, State/ Province ____________ Postal Code __________

Phone ________________ FAX ________________ E-mail ______________

Total No. of Section 1 Answers Correct ________ Incorrect ________

Method of Payment:

Check ________ VISA ________ MasterCard ________ American Express ________

Exp.Date ________

Credit Card Number:

____

Credit Card Signature:

____

I certify that I have completed this CME activity as designed.

Signature:

____

CME APPLICATION FOR UNITS IN OCCUPATIONAL AND ENVIRONMENTAL MEDICINE: SELF- ASSESSMENT REVIEW

To earn fifteen (15) CMEs of Category 1 credit toward the Physician's Recognition Award of the American Medical Association for the study of sections in *A Practical Approach to Occupational and Environmental Medicine, Second Edition,* and *Occupational and Environmental Medicine: Self-Assessment Review,* do the following:

- Study the Unit(s) in *A Practical Approach to Occupational and Environmental Medicine, Second Edition.*
- Study all of the materials in *Occupational and Environmental Medicine: Self-Assessment Review* for the corresponding Unit.
- Complete the self-test for the corresponding Unit
- Evaluate your responses by using the key at the bottom of the answer sheet. Note your score on the form.
- Complete the CME registration form and mail it with a $75 application fee (per unit) or $375 for all five sections made payable to ACOEM to:

    The Department of Education
    CME Coordinator
    The American College of Occupational and Environmental Medicine
    55 West Seegers Road
    Arlington Heights, IL 60005-3919

CME Registration for Unit 2 of
Occupational and Environmental Medicine: Self-Assessment Review
Please print clearly.

Name ____ Medical Degree ________

Address _______________ City, State/ Province ____________ Postal Code __________

Phone ________________ FAX ________________ E-mail ______________

Total No. of Section 2 Answers Correct ________ Incorrect ________

Method of Payment:

Check ________ VISA ________ MasterCard ________ American Express ________

Exp.Date ________

Credit Card Number:

____

Credit Card Signature:

____

I certify that I have completed this CME activity as designed.

Signature:

____

CME APPLICATION FOR UNITS IN OCCUPATIONAL AND ENVIRONMENTAL MEDICINE: SELF- ASSESSMENT REVIEW

To earn fifteen (15) CMEs of Category 1 credit toward the Physician's Recognition Award of the American Medical Association for the study of sections in *A Practical Approach to Occupational and Environmental Medicine, Second Edition,* and *Occupational and Environmental Medicine: Self-Assessment Review,* do the following:

- Study the Unit(s) in *A Practical Approach to Occupational and Environmental Medicine, Second Edition.*
- Study all of the materials in *Occupational and Environmental Medicine: Self-Assessment Review* for the corresponding Unit.
- Complete the self-test for the corresponding Unit
- Evaluate your responses by using the key at the bottom of the answer sheet. Note your score on the form.
- Complete the CME registration form and mail it with a $75 application fee (per unit) or $375 for all five sections made payable to ACOEM to:

    The Department of Education
    CME Coordinator
    The American College of Occupational and Environmental Medicine
    55 West Seegers Road
    Arlington Heights, IL 60005-3919

CME Registration for Unit 3 of
Occupational and Environmental Medicine: Self-Assessment Review
Please print clearly.

Name ____ Medical Degree ________

Address ________________ City, State/ Province ___________ Postal Code __________

Phone ________________ FAX ________________ E-mail ______________

Total No. of Section 3 Answers Correct ________ Incorrect ________

Method of Payment:

Check ________ VISA ________ MasterCard ________ American Express ________

Exp.Date ________

Credit Card Number:

____

Credit Card Signature:

____

I certify that I have completed this CME activity as designed.

Signature

____

CME APPLICATION FOR UNITS IN OCCUPATIONAL AND ENVIRONMENTAL MEDICINE: SELF- ASSESSMENT REVIEW

To earn fifteen (15) CMEs of Category 1 credit toward the Physician's Recognition Award of the American Medical Association for the study of sections in *A Practical Approach to Occupational and Environmental Medicine, Second Edition,* and *Occupational and Environmental Medicine: Self-Assessment Review,* do the following:

- Study the Unit(s) in *A Practical Approach to Occupational and Environmental Medicine, Second Edition.*
- Study all of the materials in *Occupational and Environmental Medicine: Self-Assessment Review* for the corresponding Unit.
- Complete the self-test for the corresponding Unit
- Evaluate your responses by using the key at the bottom of the answer sheet. Note your score on the form.
- Complete the CME registration form and mail it with a $75 application fee (per unit) or $375 for all five sections made payable to ACOEM to:

> The Department of Education
> CME Coordinator
> The American College of Occupational and Environmental Medicine
> 55 West Seegers Road
> Arlington Heights, IL 60005-3919

CME Registration for Unit 4 of
Occupational and Environmental Medicine: Self-Assessment Review
Please print clearly.

Name ____ Medical Degree ______

Address ____________________ City, State/ Province ___________ Postal Code __________

Phone ________________ FAX ________________ E-mail ______________

Total No. of Section 4 Answers Correct ______ Incorrect ______

Method of Payment:

Check ______ VISA ______ MasterCard ______ American Express ______

Exp.Date ______

Credit Card Number:

____

Credit Card Signature:

____

I certify that I have completed this CME activity as designed.

Signature:

____

CME APPLICATION FOR UNITS IN OCCUPATIONAL AND ENVIRONMENTAL MEDICINE: SELF- ASSESSMENT REVIEW

To earn fifteen (15) CMEs of Category 1 credit toward the Physician's Recognition Award of the American Medical Association for the study of sections in *A Practical Approach to Occupational and Environmental Medicine, Second Edition,* and *Occupational and Environmental Medicine: Self-Assessment Review,* do the following:

- Study the Unit(s) in *A Practical Approach to Occupational and Environmental Medicine, Second Edition.*
- Study all of the materials in *Occupational and Environmental Medicine: Self-Assessment Review* for the corresponding Unit.
- Complete the self-test for the corresponding Unit
- Evaluate your responses by using the key at the bottom of the answer sheet. Note your score on the form.
- Complete the CME registration form and mail it with a $75 application fee (per unit) or $375 for all five sections made payable to ACOEM to:

    The Department of Education
    CME Coordinator
    The American College of Occupational and Environmental Medicine
    55 West Seegers Road
    Arlington Heights, IL 60005-3919

CME Registration for Unit 5 of
Occupational and Environmental Medicine: Self-Assessment Review
Please print clearly.

Name ____ Medical Degree ________

Address ____________________ City, State/ Province ____________ Postal Code __________

Phone ____________________ FAX ____________________ E-mail ________________

Total No. of Section 5 Answers Correct ________ Incorrect ________

Method of Payment:

Check ________ VISA ________ MasterCard ________ American Express ________

Exp.Date ________

Credit Card Number:

____

Credit Card Signature:

____

I certify that I have completed this CME activity as designed.

Signature:

____

CME APPLICATION FOR UNITS IN OCCUPATIONAL AND ENVIRONMENTAL MEDICINE: SELF- ASSESSMENT REVIEW

To earn fifteen (15) CMEs of Category 1 credit toward the Physician's Recognition Award of the American Medical Association for the study of sections in *A Practical Approach to Occupational and Environmental Medicine, Second Edition,* and *Occupational and Environmental Medicine: Self-Assessment Review,* do the following:

- Study the Unit(s) in *A Practical Approach to Occupational and Environmental Medicine, Second Edition.*
- Study all of the materials in *Occupational and Environmental Medicine: Self-Assessment Review* for the corresponding Unit.
- Complete the self-test for the corresponding Unit
- Evaluate your responses by using the key at the bottom of the answer sheet. Note your score on the form.
- Complete the CME registration form and mail it with a $75 application fee (per unit) or $375 for all five sections made payable to ACOEM to:

The Department of Education
CME Coordinator
The American College of Occupational and Environmental Medicine
55 West Seegers Road
Arlington Heights, IL 60005-3919

OCCUPATIONAL AND ENVIRONMENTAL MEDICINE: SELF-ASSESSMENT REVIEW EVALUATION

Please check all that apply:

- **Resident** ☐

- **Fellow** ☐

- **Attending** ☐

- **Private Practice** ☐

- **Corporate** ☐

Years in Practice _______________________________

Specialty _______________________________

Sub-Specialty _______________________________

As a result of reading this material, will the way you manage patients change?

Yes _______________________________ No _______________________________

Comments:

Do you believe that the material was free of bias?

Yes _______________________________ No _______________________________

Comments:

Please rate:	**Excellent**			**Poor**	
Content	5	4	3	2	1
Relevance to your practice	5	4	3	2	1
CME process	5	4	3	2	1

We would appreciate your comments on the effectiveness of this learning experience. *Comments*:

Please provide suggestions for possible future programs:

ANSWER SHEET FORM
for Unit 1 in *Occupational and Environmental Medicine: Self-Assessment Review*
(Return for CME Credit Hours)

<u>Chapter 1</u>
Question 1 _________
Question 2 _________
Question 3 _________
Question 4 _________
Question 5 _________

<u>Chapter 2</u>
Question 1 _________
Question 2 _________
Question 3 _________
Question 4 _________
Question 5 _________
Question 6 _________

<u>Chapter 3</u>
Question 1 _________
Question 2 _________
Question 3 _________
Question 4 _________
Question 5 _________
Question 6 _________

<u>Chapter 4</u>
Question 1 _________
Question 2 _________
Question 3 _________
Question 4 _________
Question 5 _________
Question 6 _________

<u>Chapter 5</u>
Question 1 _________
Question 2 _________
Question 3 _________
Question 4 _________
Question 5 _________
Question 6 _________
Question 7 _________
Question 8 _________

<u>Chapter 6</u>
Question 1 _________
Question 2 _________
Question 3 _________
Question 4 _________
Question 5 _________
Question 6 _________

<u>Chapter 7</u>
Question 1 _________
Question 2 _________
Question 3 _________
Question 4 _________
Question 5 _________
Question 6 _________
Question 7 _________

<u>Chapter 8</u>
Question 1 _________
Question 2 _________
Question 3 _________
Question 4 _________
Question 5 _________
Question 6 _________

<u>Chapter 9</u>
Question 1 _________
Question 2 _________
Question 3 _________
Question 4 _________
Question 5 _________
Question 6 _________
Question 7 _________

<u>Chapter 10</u>
Question 1 _________
Question 2 _________
Question 3 _________
Question 4 _________
Question 5 _________
Question 6 _________
Question 7 _________

ANSWER SHEET FORM
for Unit 2 in *Occupational and Environmental Medicine: Self-Assessment Review*
(Return for CME Credit Hours)

<table>
<tr><td valign="top">

Chapter 11
Question 1   ________
Question 2   ________
Question 3   ________
Question 4   ________
Question 5   ________

Chapter 12
Question 1   ________
Question 2   ________
Question 3   ________
Question 4   ________

Chapter 13
Question 1   ________
Question 2   ________
Question 3   ________
Question 4   ________
Question 5   ________

Chapter 14
Question 1   ________
Question 2   ________
Question 3   ________
Question 4   ________

Chapter 15
Question 1   ________
Question 2   ________
Question 3   ________
Question 4   ________
Question 5   ________

Chapter 16
Question 1   ________
Question 2   ________
Question 3   ________
Question 4   ________

Chapter 17
Question 1   ________
Question 2   ________
Question 3   ________
Question 4   ________
Question 5   ________

</td><td valign="top">

Chapter 18
Question 1   ________
Question 2   ________
Question 3   ________
Question 4   ________

Chapter 19
Question 1   ________
Question 2   ________
Question 3   ________
Question 4   ________
Question 5   ________

Chapter 20
Question 1   ________
Question 2   ________
Question 3   ________
Question 4   ________

</td></tr>
</table>

ANSWER SHEET FORM
for Unit 3 in *Occupational and Environmental Medicine: Self-Assessment Review*
(Return for CME Credit Hours)

<u>Chapter 21</u>
Question 1 ________
Question 2 ________
Question 3 ________
Question 4 ________
Question 5 ________

<u>Chapter 22</u>
Question 1 ________
Question 2 ________
Question 3 ________
Question 4 ________
Question 5 ________
Question 6 ________
Question 7 ________

<u>Chapter 23</u>
Question 1 ________
Question 2 ________
Question 3 ________
Question 4 ________
Question 5 ________

<u>Chapter 24</u>
Question 1 ________
Question 2 ________
Question 3 ________
Question 4 ________
Question 5 ________
Question 6 ________

<u>Chapter 25</u>
Question 1 ________
Question 2 ________
Question 3 ________
Question 4 ________
Question 5 ________

<u>Chapter 26</u>
Question 1 ________
Question 2 ________
Question 3 ________
Question 4 ________

<u>Chapter 27</u>
Question 1 ________
Question 2 ________
Question 3 ________

<u>Chapter 28</u>
Question 1 ________
Question 2 ________
Question 3 ________
Question 4 ________
Question 5 ________

<u>Chapter 29</u>
Question 1 ________
Question 2 ________
Question 3 ________
Question 4 ________

<u>Chapter 30</u>
Question 1 ________
Question 2 ________
Question 3 ________
Question 4 ________
Question 5 ________

Chapter 31
Question 1 ________
Question 2 ________
Question 3 ________
Question 4 ________
Question 5 ________
Question 6 ________
Question 7 ________
Question 8 ________

Chapter 32
Question 1 ________
Question 2 ________
Question 3 ________
Question 4 ________
Question 5 ________

Chapter 33
Question 1 ________
Question 2 ________
Question 3 ________
Question 4 ________
Question 5 ________

Chapter 34
Question 1 ________
Question 2 ________
Question 3 ________
Question 4 ________
Question 5 ________
Question 6 ________

Chapter 35
Question 1 ________
Question 2 ________
Question 3 ________
Question 4 ________
Question 5 ________
Question 6 ________

Chapter 36
Question 1 ________
Question 2 ________
Question 3 ________
Question 4 ________

Chapter 37
Question 1 ________
Question 2 ________
Question 3 ________
Question 4 ________
Question 5 ________
Question 6 ________
Question 7 ________

Chapter 38
Question 1 ________
Question 2 ________
Question 3 ________
Question 4 ________
Question 5 ________
Question 6 ________
Question 7 ________

Chapter 39
Question 1 ________
Question 2 ________
Question 3 ________
Question 4 ________
Question 5 ________
Question 6 ________
Question 7 ________
Question 8 ________

Chapter 40
Question 1 ________
Question 2 ________
Question 3 ________
Question 4 ________
Question 5 ________

ANSWER SHEET FORM
for Unit 5 in *Occupational and Environmental Medicine: Self-Assessment Review*
(Return for CME Credit Hours)

<table>
<tr><td valign="top">

Chapter 41
Question 1 ________
Question 2 ________
Question 3 ________
Question 4 ________
Question 5 ________

Chapter 42
Question 1 ________
Question 2 ________
Question 3 ________
Question 4 ________
Question 5 ________

Chapter 43
Question 1 ________
Question 2 ________
Question 3 ________
Question 4 ________

Chapter 44
Question 1 ________
Question 2 ________
Question 3 ________
Question 4 ________
Question 5 ________

Chapter 45
Question 1 ________
Question 2 ________
Question 3 ________
Question 4 ________

Chapter 46
Question 1 ________
Question 2 ________
Question 3 ________
Question 4 ________

Chapter 47
Question 1 ________
Question 2 ________
Question 3 ________
Question 4 ________
Question 5 ________

Chapter 48
Question 1 ________
Question 2 ________
Question 3 ________
Question 4 ________

</td><td valign="top">

Chapter 49
Question 1 ________
Question 2 ________
Question 3 ________

Chapter 50
Question 1 ________
Question 2 ________
Question 3 ________
Question 4 ________
Question 5 ________

</td></tr>
</table>

Learning and Performance Strategies for the Occupational Medicine Certification Examination

Certification and recertification processes are intended to ensure that practitioners maintain their competence. When you take the occupational medicine board examination, you are evaluating your clinical knowledge and comparing yourself with your peers. When you recertify, you are satisfying yourself, your colleagues, and your patients that you have continued to keep up to date. Because certification and recertification scores tend to be the strongest predictors of subsequent recertification scores (1,2), it is important to maximize your knowledge and your test-taking skills early in your career.

As a physician, you have achieved numerous academic milestones in your life. Successfully completing undergraduate education, medical school, and one or more postgraduate programs means that you have taken many formal examinations. In your early years of academic training, and perhaps during the academic portion of your residency training, examinations were frequent throughout courses. Although at the time you may not have looked at it this way, frequent tests are actually motivating and informative; they provide feedback concerning how well you are succeeding at mastering content, and they guide your future study. In your clinical practice years, it is typical that the only formal examinations you experience are the certification examinations for your specialty or specialties. Once certified in occupational medicine, you will sit for recertification in ten years.

When you experience long intervals between examinations, test-preparation and test-taking skills you once used automatically may no longer be immediately available to you. This section will acquaint you with information about effective approaches to learning in general, as well as some specific advice about preparing for and taking the occupational medicine certification examination. As you read, try to recall specific techniques that have worked well for you in the past. Jot down your ideas so that you can use them in your current preparation. You can also keep a record for future use.

ORGANIZING FOR LEARNING

Where do you currently work when you are studying? Do you have an organized area in which you keep resources and the written products you create as you learn? Committing or recommitting a place devoted exclusively to studying can enhance your learning sessions. To determine an appropriate selection of study materials, consult Meyer's list of resources in this volume, and the list of materials provided in the "Study Guide Materials/Exam Content Outlines from the American Board of Preventive Medicine" (3). In addition, for a recommended approach to reading to maintain competence in any medical specialty, see the chapter by Sackett et al., "Surveying the

Medical Literature to Keep Up to Date in Clinical Epidemiology: A Basic Science for Clinical Medicine" (4). The authors offer a comprehensive method for selecting and reviewing pertinent literature.

According to studies of experts and novices in fields such as physics and medicine, not only do experts have more knowledge than novices, but their knowledge is also better organized and developed (5). As you study, notice the categories of information that are easy for you to remember as opposed to those that take more effort. It's likely that easy-to-recall information is well learned and well organized in your memory. You will need to work at learning (often relearning) more difficult information and organizing it for rapid recall. You will probably need to spend more time and effort on these latter categories.

Because learning tasks are not all of the same difficulty level, you will want to choose times at which you have the greatest ability to focus to perform the most demanding work. Reading and taking notes requires intense concentration, so you can target times at which you're most alert and unlikely to be distracted for such tasks. To get the most from these intensive sessions, 1) review what you mastered in your most recent study session; 2) create a written product as you learn new material, in your own words or design (such as an outline, matrix or diagram); and 3) decide what and when you will study next.

The less demanding tasks of reviewing and practicing what you've mastered in your intensive sessions can be fit in at other times. On breaks at work or at home, or perhaps while you re walking, riding in a car, or waiting in line at a bank or store, challenge yourself to re-produce information, rather than passively re-viewing it. Discussing study topics with colleagues, residents, or students, informally or as part of a structured study group (for example, a journal club), can also reinforce your learning.

PREPARING FOR THE EXAMINATION

Educational researchers have investigated a number of approaches to preparing for examinations and recommend an approach consisting of assessing your current capacity to perform on the examination, acquiring new material, encoding new material and developing cues for retention, reviewing, and maintaining motivation (6):

Assess Your Current Capacity to Perform on the Exam

To effectively plan and use study time, familiarize yourself with the content and the format of the occupational medicine certification examination. A content outline is provided in the pamphlet "Study Guide Materials/Exam Content Outlines" provided by the American Board of Preventive Medicine (3). Knowing your current level of knowledge in each content area can help you determine how best to schedule your learning sessions—the frequency and duration of study times you'll need. For example, use the self-test in this book to determine which subjects need the most effort, and then apportion the time for studying accordingly. Because we know that goal-setting facilitates learning, it will benefit you to write out a master study schedule with a specific topic or topics designated for each study period. Do this in pencil so that you can make adjustments as needed. After all, once you delve into a subject you may learn that you know more or less than you estimated.

Of course, your experience in the clinic also informs you about your current knowledge level. When in your daily work you find yourself needing to look up information or consult with a colleague, you have an insight into an area on which you may need to focus in a study session. Try jotting down questions that arise during the day, and then follow up by writing out the answers you find and adding this information to your existing study materials.

In addition to familiarizing yourself with exam content, you will want to know what to expect with respect to test format. The American Board of Preventive Medicine pamphlet mentioned above provides a description of the test as well as sample questions. Because answering examination questions methodically and efficiently increases feelings of confidence and control during the exam, be sure to practice answering questions during each of your study sessions, or at least once or twice a week. Practice makes the process seem automatic, so answering questions will demand less mental energy and time during the actual test.

Some physicians find it worthwhile to create and take one or more mock examinations that are representative of the certification exam. Simulating the actual exam setting and time allotment, or even giving yourself less time than you will have to complete the test, can inform you about your ability to progress through the actual test. The purpose of such rehearsal is to make the certification examination seem like a familiar experience.

Acquire New Material

Reading is the most common method for acquiring new information. Because reading can be both effortful and time-consuming, it's important to use this skill strategically. This means carefully pinpointing exactly which material needs to be processed in depth versus that which can be skimmed or skipped entirely. Too often, we revert to the habit of starting with the first word in a chapter or article and reading every word until we reach the end or until we find that we have lost concentration. Use your reading time efficiently. "Shop" for precisely the information you need and no more. Ask yourself, "Exactly what do I want to be able to say or write when I've finished reading this?" Then search for that information.

When using study guides in which pre-tests and post-tests are provided, use the questions at the beginning of each unit to target your reading, then select only the information that needs attention. On the post-test, skip questions unrelated to your reading. Use the table of contents and index of a book to help you determine exactly which chapters, and which sections within them, to read. Once you've selected what to read, get a structural overview by glancing at the introductory material, scanning through headings and boldfaced or italicized words, and noting any summaries that are provided. For some topics, this approach alone will provide everything you need to know. Journal articles can be approached in the same way. Ask yourself what new information you wish to gain by reading the article. Scan the article to determine its structure and then read only the sections that contribute new knowledge or understanding to your current knowledge.

Encode New Material and Develop Cues for Retention

Once you've identified and understood information to add to your knowledge base, you want to ensure that you'll retain it. Too often, after the hard work of reading and understanding, we simply shelve reading material and trust that we ll be able to remember what we read. As time goes by, memory fades, and we eventually find ourselves looking for the same information again.

Notetaking allows you to structure and save information that you want to store both in your long-term memory and in your external memory—your written files and notecards, for example. With some articles or other printed matter that you intend to keep on file, underlining or highlighting information may be sufficient. However, be aware that these activities are simply recognition techniques. In other words, you've designated the data that you want to know, but often you haven't processed it enough to master it.

For information you want to make your own, you need to do more than underline or highlight. You might write a summary sentence or notes at the top of an article or on the first page of a chapter you're saving. However, to truly integrate and own new knowledge, you may need to produce separate cards or pages on which you create written or graphical memory aids. Sackett et al. recommend encoding an article's key details on a 3 in. x 5 in. card and keeping it in your pocket until you have committed the new knowledge to memory (4). Another method is to create flash cards with a term, concept, or question on one side and the answer or explanation on the reverse. Some learners create a split-page note-taking system that mimics flash cards: they write the term or question on the left-hand side of a page and record the explanation on the right. They then can lay pages of notes atop one another, with only the question columns showing, and quiz themselves. Flash cards or split-page notetaking allows you to actively test yourself on recently mastered material to make sure you are retaining it. These methods force you to ask yourself questions about what you've studied, rather than simply "re-viewing" notes on a written page—a passive and often ineffective study method.

More complex memory devices include outlines, summaries, matrices, diagrams, algorithms, and concept maps. All of these but the last are familiar memory aids. A concept map is a newer idea and is a graphical method of demonstrating both the elements of information in a conceptual network and the relationships among them (7). While concept maps deal with cognitive information, the fact that they represent it visually takes advantage of the fact that concrete visual information is usually remembered better than abstract or conceptual information (5). A concept map has been included at the end of this section.

Just as concept maps help us to remember because of their visual presentation, mnemonic devices assist us in remembering because they provide cues for retrieval of information that we wish to remember. For example, the acronym PINES assists one to remember the differential diagnosis for a chest x-ray with a reticulonodular pattern: pneumoconiosis, infection (e.g., miliary tuberculosis), neoplasm, (e.g., alveolar cell cancer), eosinophilic granuloma, and sarcoidosis. Similarly, two mnemonics are used in remembering symptoms of organophosphate poisoning. DUMBELS refers to the muscarinic effects of defecation, urination, miosis, bronchospasm/bradycardia, emesis, lacrimation, and salivation/sweating. Nicotinic effects are remembered using MATCH—muscle weakness/fasiculations, adrenal medulla activity, tachycardia, cramping of skeletal muscles, and hypertension.

Review

Taking the steps outlined above in order to locate, understand, and organize knowledge is usually quite a thought- and labor-intensive process. In order to ensure that this hard work pays off in practice and on the board examination, an additional step is required. Once you have mastered information, spaced review is necessary to promote recall in the future.

Memory researchers have found that memory performance improves with repeated attempts at recall. On a regular basis, challenge yourself to re-produce information that you have previously learned. To enhance memory, elaborate in more than one way on the information you're refreshing (8). For example, draw a concept map or create a diagram in addition to stating aloud or writing the targeted information. A weekly review of newly mastered knowledge is recommended, followed by intermittent reviews.

An additional memory-enhancing principle is overlearning, which is continued learning beyond the point of simple mastery. Education researchers have demonstrated that overlearning strengthens learning and improves retrieval speed.

Maintain Motivation

Occupational physicians are motivated to pass the certification examination for many reasons. Being certified is a key career goal which leads to job opportunity and to personal and professional satisfaction. For many physicians, the examination process is an emotional experience. Wlodkowski, who has written extensively on adults' motivation, points out that because adult learning often deals with success and failure in achievement and accomplishment activities, learners often react quite emotionally to their progress or lack of it. He emphasizes that an adult's emotional state is a significant influence on learning. Wlodkowski further notes that emotions not only influence behavior but may affect thinking as well. Therefore, he recommends that adults work to maintain a positive attitude toward learning, which can in turn assist them to persist at learning and also deepen their interest in the material that they are studying (9).

Reminding yourself of your professional goals and how your knowledge mastery and subsequent certification and/or recertification fits in with your lifetime career plans can be motivating. For example, Meyer (this volume) suggests that physicians reflect upon and appreciate the satisfaction that comes from completing an organized review of one's field, the confidence that results from knowing that knowledge gaps have been addressed, and the improvement in teaching that can accompany content mastery. It is also likely that you will note a positive impact on your clinical practice from your studying, and this can be a source of regular reinforcement for your efforts.

The learning processes suggested in this chapter are recommended by education researchers and learning specialists to be effective in helping you to reach your goals of keeping up to date and becoming board certified or recertified. However, these processes are also complex and time consuming. To help you to persist, Wlodkowski recommends that you consider including some of the following features in your study program: using a variety of materials from which to study; keeping your study materials in an organized, orderly fashion; breaking large topics into small, manageable chunks; and spending some time in group study (9).

Wlodkowski notes that a sense of competence occurs when an adult realizes that he or she has achieved personal mastery. While the end goal of the certification process is to obtain the professional recognition of mastery, you can create a sense of personal mastery in the interim by tracking your performance throughout your study sessions. Once you have determined the subject matters you need to focus on, consider creating a graph, chart, or narrative journal through which you document your progress. Log the nature and amount of reading you do, for example, and count the number of note cards or note pages you produce. Examining this documentation and reflecting upon your learning strategies can provide insights about those techniques that are paying off and should be retained, and those that are inefficient and could be altered or abandoned. When testing yourself, chart how many questions you attempt in a subject area and the percentage you answer correctly. You can increase both your confidence level and your motivation to persist by providing feedback for yourself that informs you about how well you are doing and allows you to make internal statements such as "I really understand this", or "I am doing proficiently" (9).

TAKING THE EXAMINATION

Meyer, in this volume, provides comprehensive information about the occupational certification examination itself, and he suggests many practical strategies for approaching the trip to the exam site and the experience of taking the exam. His advice corresponds with that of many experienced test-takers who have found that having a game plan for the examination allows them to feel calmer and in better control. Some additional suggestions follow.

- At the examination itself, as soon as you are permitted to open your test booklet, open to a blank page and write out any information you think you may forget under the pressure of the examination, such as mnemonic devices, outlines, or other memory aids that you have developed in preparation for the test. Some physicians have found that even jotting down points that may seem easy to recall actually saves time later. This step can help you easily remember your memory devices so you do not have to take time to access them while you're focusing on test content. One occupational medicine physician wrote out formulas and sketched out blank two-by-two tables before starting the test. She noted that having them at hand was helpful because you can get caught up in the wording of the problem and you don't think about what you're really looking at in tables, diagrams, etc.

- Next, read the directions and survey the test. Some of the most important reading you'll do is in the directions, rather than in the questions. Be certain that you understand directions thoroughly and follow them to the letter. To use time effectively, an important next step is to survey the test. This way you can find out where the lengthy or challenging problems are, and plan your time accordingly. You do not have to answer questions in the order in which they appear. Choose the most logical order for yourself. Some people prefer to answer easy questions first to gain confidence. Others find that difficult questions prey on their mind and distract them, so they address those first. When answering questions out of order, it is essential, of course, to be meticulous about answering each question in its appropriate location on the answer sheet.
- Some physicians find it helpful to sketch out a time schedule for the entire morning or afternoon session. They can judge their progress against this estimate in order be able to answer all of the questions and save time for checking that they have marked their answers correctly. Another helpful technique to pace yourself appropriately is to mark the half-way spot in the test booklet and check the time at which you arrive there. You may find that you need to speed up in order to finish.
- As you answer questions, work at a quick, steady pace. Keep your place on your answer sheet with your pencil and move it methodically as you advance through the test. For multiple choice questions, try reading only the "stem", or leading statement, of the question, think about what you know about the topic, and then predict the answer. This way you can look among the choices and find the answer you predicted, rather than being distracted by choices that may seem plausible as you consider them. If you can't predict an answer, examine the choices, eliminate those that you can, and guess. You may prefer to reserve your final choice until later. In either case, make a mark in the test margin so that you can return to the question. After more experience with the test, you may find the question easier to answer. Of course, since all answers are of equal value, you will want to avoid lingering on difficult questions, and you will want to answer every question.
- Narrative questions require careful, focused reading. A helpful approach is to scan the questions before reading the passage so that you can eliminate unnecessary information as you read—you might even draw a line through irrelevant facts so that you won't reread them. Some physicians like to underline key points or create an abstract or outline on the side of the passage so that they can collect facts as they read. They then refer only to these notes, without having to go back to the narrative.
- A final point is to continue to stay aware of the time as you progress through the test. You will want to save five to ten minutes at the end of each session to check to make sure that you have recorded your answers accurately.

Once the test is over, reflect upon your test-preparation and test-taking experience. Record insights about content that you knew well, as well as content that was more challenging than you expected. Note the examination-preparation and test-taking strategies that you found useful and will want to repeat, as well as those that should be revised. After all, if all goes as well as you expect, you will not be taking another certification examination for ten years, and at that time you may be grateful that you have a file that can guide you through another successful certification experience.

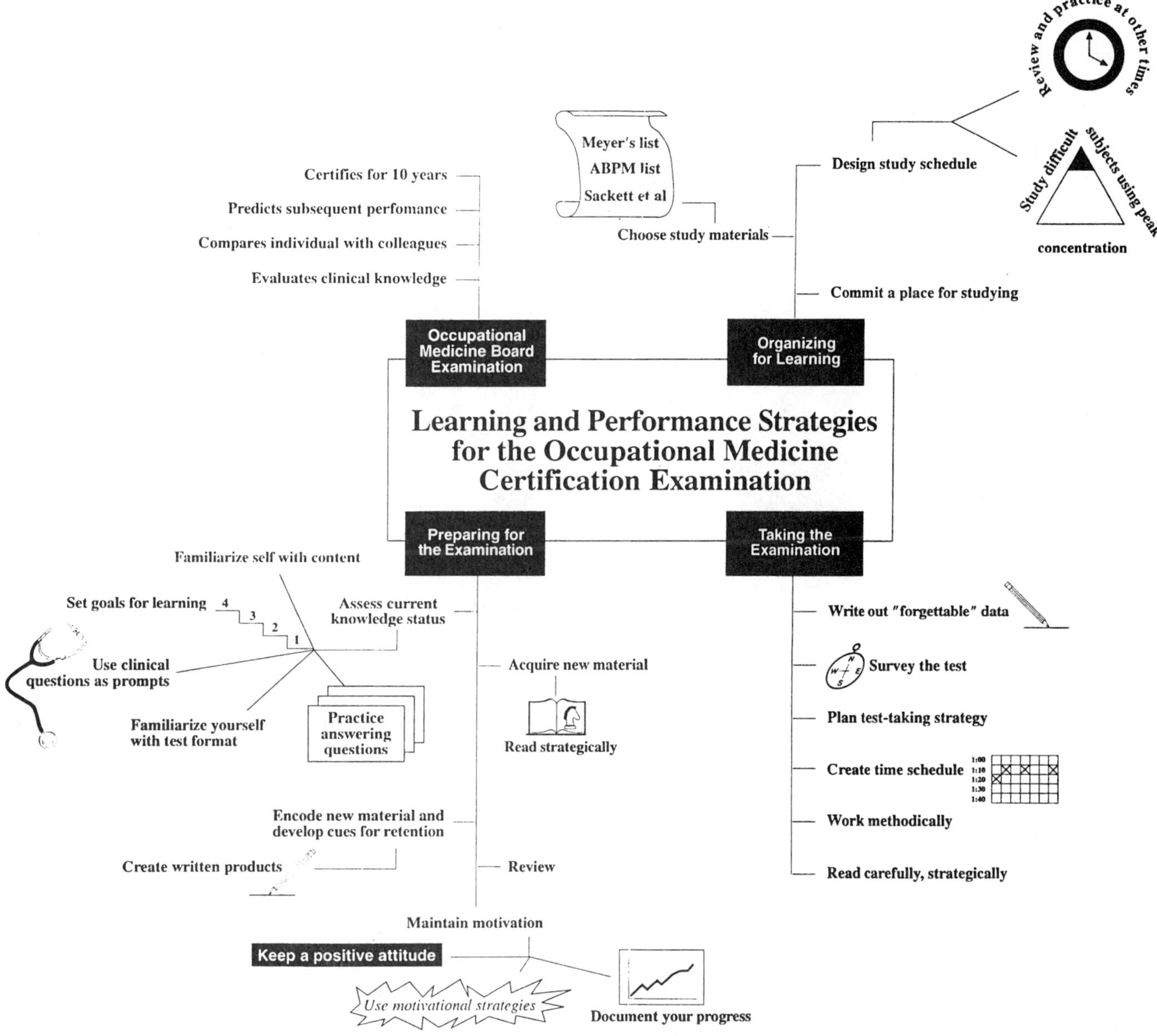

Figure 1. A concept map of the preceding section.

REFERENCES

1. Leigh, T.M., Johnson, T.P., and Piscano, N.J. Predictive validity of the American Board of Family Practice in-training examination. *Acad Med* 1990;65:454.
2. Waxman, H., Braunstein, G., Dantzker, D., et al. Performance on the internal medicine second-year residency in-training examination predicts the outcome of the ABIM certifying examination. *J Gen Intern Med* 1994;9:692.
3. Study guide materials/Exam content outlines. American Board of Preventive Medicine, Inc.
4. Sackett, D.L., Haynes, R.B., Guyatt, G.H., and Tugwell, P. *Clinical Epidemiology: A Basic Science for Clinical Medicine (2nd ed.)*. Boston: Little Brown, 1991.
5. Pressley, M. and El-Dinary, P.B. Memory Strategy Instruction that Promotes Good Information Processing. In: D.J. Hermann, H. Weingartner, A. Searleman, and C. McEvoy (eds.), *Memory Improvement: Implications for Memory Theory*. New York: Springer-Verlag, 1992.

6. Flippo, R.F. and Caverly, D.C. (eds.). *Teaching Reading and Study Strategies at the College Level*. Newark, Delaware: International Reading Association, 1991.
7. Glynn, S.M., Yeany, R.H., and Britton, B.K. (eds.). *The Psychology Of Learning Science*. Hillsdale, NJ: Lawrence Erlbaum Associates, 1991.
8. Hermann, D.J., Weingartner, H., Searleman, A., and McEvoy, C. (eds.). *Memory Improvement: Implications for Memory Theory*. New York: Springer-Verlag, 1992.
9. Wlodkowski, R.J. *Enhancing Adult Motivation to Learn: A Guide to Improving Instruction and Increasing Learner Achievement*. San Francisco: Jossey-Bass, 1991.

Linda M. Roth, Ph.D.

Taking the Board Exam in Occupational Medicine

The American Board of Preventive Medicine (ABPM) offers certification in the specialties of Occupational Medicine, Aerospace Medicine, and General Preventive Medicine based on the results of an examination given in November of each year. Eligibility to sit for the examination is determined by criteria set forth by the Board, and is based upon residency training and practice in the field, or on several alternate pathways for those who graduated from medical school before widespread training in the field was available. Requirements for admission to the exam, as well as application forms, are available from the Board at the address listed at the end of this section. This section provides principles for review and study for the board examination. Increased familiarity with strategies for review will increase the likelihood of a passing score. Used in conjunction with this study guide, this section will help to give a prospective examinee a clearer picture of how to systematically acquire the knowledge base for both passing the certification exam and for subsequent practice in occupational medicine.

THE ABPM EXAM: SCOPE AND CONTENT

The ABPM examination is a full-day, seven-hour exam given in two parts. The core examination, which covers preventive medicine as a whole (including basic questions on each of the three specialty areas), consists of 250 multiple-choice questions. Four hours are allotted for completion of the morning core section. The afternoon is devoted to specialty exams in occupational, aerospace, and preventive medicine; three hours are given to complete this 150-question section. A passing score is required on both morning and afternoon sections of the exam for certification in Preventive Medicine. The pass rate for the exam varies from year to year based upon the Board's assessment of the distribution of scores for that year, but in general two-thirds or less of examinees are certified yearly in occupational medicine. According to statistics provided by the Board, the overall pass rate in 1995 was 72% for the ABPM examinations; 65% of examinees passed the occupational medicine boards. The failure rate on the exam is therefore substantial. Thorough preparation, beginning four to six months before the boards, is required in order to have a chance at a passing score.

The material that appears on the core and specialty exams is outlined in a pamphlet prepared by the ABPM (Tables 1 and 2). The core section tests the examinee's knowledge of epidemiology, biostatistics, preventive health services and administration, environmental health, and behavioral factors in preventive medicine, as well as basic information related to the three specialty areas. Although the content of the core section may change slightly every year, biostatistics and epidemiology are certain to be covered in detail, and a thorough grounding in these areas is essential to pass the morning session. The afternoon exam in occupational medicine covers material on the worker and the workplace, occupational toxicology, occupational medical management, clinical occupational medicine, and physical and biological hazards of the workplace.

TABLE 1. *Exam Content Outline, Core Examination*

I. Administration
   A. Policy development and management
   B. Administration principles and applications
II. Biostatistics
   A. Design and methods
   B. Interpretation and applications
   C. Vital statistics and demography
III. Clinical
   A. Acute
   B. Chronic
   C. Genetic
   D. Maternal and Child Health
   E. Occupational
   F. Alternative types of care
IV. Epidemiology
   A. Design and methods
   B. Interpretation
   C. Determinants of disease
   D. Prevention and control
   E. Legal and ethical issues
V. Behavioral
   A. Health education and promotion (group)
   B. Lifestyle (individual)
VI. Environmental
   A. Agents
   B. Community health
   C. Industrial health and safety
   D. Legal issues

REVIEWING: WHAT TO STUDY

Clearly, no single source can provide all the material needed to prepare for and pass the board exam in occupational medicine. In studying for the exam, plan to use a number of reference sources, each with its own particular strengths. For the core section of the boards, the texts that have stood the tests of time and usefulness are the Maxcy-Rosenau-Last *Public Health and Preventive Medicine,* now in its 13th edition, and Brett Cassens' outline and study guide *Preventive Medicine and Public Health* (see the end of this section for full citations). These texts serve particularly well for review of environmental health, health care administration, and the public health aspects of chronic disease. For epidemiology and biostatistics, many find that the single best guide is the *Study Guide to Epidemiology and Biostatistics* by Morton, Hebel, and McCarter. The time taken to master the material and study questions in this small book will be rewarded by an understanding of the material sufficient to answer nearly any epi/biostats question the board can ask. Finally, two standard public health texts that should be included in any review (and from which many exam questions appeared to be taken) are the *Guide to Clinical Preventive Services* of the U. S. Preventive Services Task Force, now in an updated 1996 edition, and Benenson's *Control of Communicable Diseases Manual*, which outlines the epidemiology and public health management of infectious diseases.

Occupational medicine texts useful for board review can be grouped into two categories: the comprehensive text used as an encyclopedic reference during training and practice, and the shorter guides to the range of occupational health problems and practice, which provide concise summaries valuable for review as study time becomes limited. In the first category are the texts by Rom, Zenz et al., and Rosenstock and Cullen. At least one of these references should be read cover-to-cover during your training or practice year to gain a thorough grounding in clinical occupational medicine; these texts can be used in much the same way that Cecil or Harrison, for example, are used in internal medicine. Among the shorter concise reviews are McCunney's *Practical*

TABLE 2. *Exam Content Outline, Occupational Medicine*

I. The Workplace
  A. Environmental assessment
  B. Ergonomics
  C. Data collection methods
  D. Record keeping and legal requirements
  E. Notification requirements
  F. Hazard control
II. The Worker
  A. Job compatibility
  B. Worker education
  C. Special considerations
  D. Disability
  E. Work/rest cycles: chronobiology
III. Occupational Medical Services
  A. Elements of services
  B. Resources and facilities
  C. Staffing, costs, budgets
  D. Governmental Services
  E. First-aid providers
  F. Disaster planning
  G. Travelers health services; tropical and third-world
     public health
IV. Occupational Medical Practice
  A. Training and certification
  B. Ethical considerations
  C. Record-keeping, automation
  D. Information disclosure, privileged communications
  E. Insurance issues
  F. Legal procedures
  G. Wellness
  H. Behavioral factors in health and illness
  I. Occupational health standards; regulations

V. Clinical Occupational Medicine
  A. Dermatology
  B. Musculoskeletal conditions
  C. Cardiopulmonary
  D. Neurology-Psychiatry
  E. Hepatic and renal function
  F. Reproduction
VI. Industrial Toxicology
  A. General Principles
  B. Experimental Toxicology
  C. Pneumoconioses
  D. Industrial hypersensitivity reactions
  E. Asphyxiants
  F. Pulmonary irritants
  G. Metals
  H. Organic compounds
  I. Chemical carcinogenesis and carcinogens
VII. Physical Hazards
  A. Noise and bioacoustics
  B. Radiation, ionizing
  C. Radiation, non-ionizing
  D. Vibration
  E. Temperature extremes, thermal injury
  F. Hyper- and hypobaric environments and dysbarism
  G. Mechanical injury
VIII. Biologic Hazards
  A. Principles of disease transfer and control
  B. Immunization techniques
  C. Disease detection
  D. Principal occupational hazards (TB, hepatitis B, HIV)
  E. Tropical diseases and prophylaxis
  F. Zoonotic infections

Guide to Occupational and Environmental Medicine, LaDou's *Occupational Medicine*, and Levy and Wegman's *Occupational Health*. All highly readable and valuable as references as you continue to practice in occupational medicine, at least two of these sources should be used to integrate material presented from different aspects of occupational medicine practice. The *ATSDR Case Studies in Environmental Medicine*, published by the U. S. Public Health Service, provide concise outlines and study questions on common environmental toxicants. Finally, it is essential to review the management aspects of occupational health, although this information is rarely covered in clinical textbooks. The material in McCunney's text, supplemented by either Moser's or Felton's monographs on OEM management, will serve to cover the details of this area. A recent issue of the *Occupational Medicine State-of-the-Art Reviews*, entitled *Law and the Workplace*, will be exceptionally useful in review of legal and regulatory issues, especially in regard to the Americans with Disabilities Act.

Several study guides which supplement and focus the material needed to review for the boards are available. This volume and the accompanying examination questions will help you to review and solidify the knowledge gained from McCunney's *Practical Approach* text. Additionally, the study guide available from the OEM press, available in a new edition this year, provides a nondirected but comprehensive review for both the core exam and all three specialty exams. Considerable effort is required to work through this guide, but for those whose manner of study it fits, it can be well worth the effort. An alternative means of exam preparation is represented in board review courses given by several organizations including the American College of Preventive Medicine. If your motivation to review is stimulated by didactic or lecture approaches, these materials can be worthwhile for those who can spare the travel and classroom time.

REVIEWING: HOW TO STUDY

Regardless of your style of study, a considerable investment of time is required to review for the exam. Preparation should begin four to six months before the scheduled exam date in early November; little can be gained and much will be forgotten or left uncovered by late cramming close to the date of the exam. Time management can be difficult, particularly for those starting the practice year in occupational medicine and faced with a host of other demands on their attention. Nonetheless, like the baseball manager's old saw that games in May are just as important as those in September, time spent consistently preparing early is likely to pay dividends as the board exam draws closer. Your areas of weakness can be identified and attended to with less hurry once the majority of material has been covered. Therefore, pick a time, even an hour or two, to review *daily*, beginning in June or earlier if possible, and stick to it religiously. Most helpful is to get into a routine when reviewing. If a particular time of day is most suitable (for example, the early morning hours before work or the evening just after the clinic has closed), make it a daily routine to read and review at that time. Early establishment of a daily study time and routine will prove a good defense against procrastination, and ensure that there is always time carved out of the day to get the work done.

Now that I've covered what to study, the question arises: *How* do you study for the Boards? For some, this exam might be the next in a long series of standardized exams dating back to the PSAT in high school, and interpreting the questions and filling in the ovals on the answer sheet may be second nature. More likely, this exam comes after at least several years spent in practice or another work setting, and the exam skills learned earlier have long since atrophied. No one will pretend that it is not hard work to regain those skills, yet taking a positive mental attitude toward doing it can have its rewards. As a physician taking a board exam late in his career wrote:

> All in all, taking a subspecialty board exam at the age of 54 was great fun. A systematic review of the literature is always worthwhile, and there is no stimulus like a formal examination to coerce a person into actually doing this. The day before the examination, I had a feeling of great mastery of a large body of knowledge, and frankly I felt as if I were 25 again. (McNamara, p. 1795)

This leads to some basic principles that can be established to increase the effectiveness of studying for an exam, namely concentration, integration, and problem-solving. Each can be outlined with respect to studying for the ABPM examination.

To effectively review this amount of material, it will be important to develop the habit of *concentration*. The location in which you study should be comfortable and as clear as possible from extraneous distractions. Most importantly, your mind should also be cleared of extraneous thoughts. Various meditative exercises can be useful in clearing your mind before study. Dr. Herbert Benson's famous series on the relaxation response describes one such technique aimed at a Western audience; students of yoga or Zen can utilize similar methods. Invariably, distracting thoughts arise when you set your mind to reading and studying. You may be wondering if you will pass the exam; you may be concerned about a patient or situation that you dealt with earlier in the day. It is important not to let these thoughts continue to deter you from your task by dwelling on them. Instead, acknowledge the thoughts that have come to you, if necessary make a note to yourself to deal with it later, and return to your study with a cleared mind. By emptying your mind of all that is extraneous to the subject in front of you at the moment, you will not only increase the power of your concentration, but you will also become less anxious about taking the examination itself.

Integration is the second principle that can be used to increase your ability to retain the material you need to learn. Different texts and different sources vary in their presentation and interpretation of the material. By being aware of differing points of view, by taking into account the differing presentations to different professionals (the clinician vs. the researcher vs. the administrator), and by asking yourself what might be missing from one text that is covered elsewhere, you can increase your knowledge of the material by correlating the information from two or three different sources. Integrate what you are learning from a variety of viewpoints and disciplines. As you review, consider what the ramifications of exposure to a hazard are from the viewpoint of the clinician, the industrial hygienist, the health services manager, the epidemiologist, and the regulator. This approach will help you to cover the specified content areas outlined by the ABPM for the exam (as noted above, they are: the worker and the workplace, occupational toxicology, occupational medical management, clinical occupational medicine, physical and biological hazards of the workplace) for a given substance or hazard. By doing this, you will establish a multi-dimensional view of a topic, and this material will be retained longer because of a greater *understanding* of the subject. A method that works for many people, is to create a system of file cards for most of the hazards you review, including metals, solvents, and pesticides. As you read, abstract material from different sources onto the card, especially information regarding the subject areas noted above. Similarly, overview cards correlating effects and hazards can be made, for example listing dermatologic effects of specific solvents. These cards can then be used for review without returning to the original texts later in the fall.

A related point is my admonition to keep your eyes and ears open at all times in your training and practice. Many things that I explored in-depth via projects in my practicum year, which at the time seemed of limited import outside of the particular question I was working on, did show up in questions on the examination. It is likely you will have the same experience; always consider what you do daily in practice and training as preparation for the exam.

Problem-solving is the last of the three aids to study. Numerous studies of learning demonstrate that direct, purposeful experience is the most powerful method by which we learn, while other forms of pedagogy make much less of an impression. We all have experienced this phenomenon in our training and practice; consider how much you learned from responsibility for direct patient care during medical school and residency as compared with the didactic teaching (often not practically reinforced) of the first two years in medical school. This method of learning can have its limitations when the need to review for a comprehensive exam arises. No one can have seen all the patients or clinical situations presented on the boards. However, in using a study guide such as this one, you can try to adopt a version of this experiential approach. Consider each question as a problem to be solved, and use the same texts, articles, and other authoritative sources that you would use when faced with a clinical or evaluative problem. Discuss the solution with peers or other knowledgeable sources if needed. Only then, once you have arrived at a solution to the problem, should you check the answer in the guide. Regular reading of periodicals, especially the *Morbidity and Mortality Weekly Reports*, will also help reinforce the principles of public health you are studying by demonstrating their application to current problems and situations. The odds are that by proceeding in this way you will explore the subject in greater depth than is provided by an answer key, and that you will retain it longer by having done so.

TAKING THE EXAM

Now that preparation for the boards has been discussed, I would also like to offer some advice about taking the exam itself. Much depends on the individual habits and style of the examinee, but a few general points can be offered. First of all, recognize that travel can be a fatiguing process, especially when balanced with the demands of work and exam preparation. I advise arriving at the site of the examination (currently in Chicago) at least a day ahead of schedule to settle into a routine in the hotel. Make sure that you can be well rested for the day of the exam. Moderate exercise can be a good stress reliever (this advice applies outside of board preparation as well) and Chicago is a superb city to visit if you need a distraction from studying. Little can be gained by an attempt to study after you have arrived, and may serve only to increase your apprehension about taking the exam. If you feel the need to review, pick no more than one or two small subjects (epidemiologic rates and ratios is one such topic) where last-minute memorization of formulas would be advantageous. Then quit studying entirely.

Knowing that you have appropriately prepared with respect to the smaller details can help reduce the stresses of exam day itself. Wear casual comfortable clothes, since you will be sitting there for most of the day. Always make certain that your entrance ticket is with you, and that you have several pencils (I brought ten, used six) available. In 1995 the testers provided individual pencil sharpeners, a small but important detail that made taking the exam easier. No food or other materials are permitted on the tabletop during the exam, however, I brought an energy bar and other small snacks to the exam to eat just before starting, and thereby staved off the drop in concentration that comes when I'm hungry. Finally, schedule your flight out for late in the day (or stay in Chicago overnight) so that time pressures of travel will not affect your performance in the afternoon section.

Keep in mind the time allotted for the examination. The morning section of the exam is the most pressured, with four hours given to answer 250 questions, which allows an average of less than a minute per question. Many examinees are unable to finish the morning section because of these time limitations. If, after you have spent a minute on a particular question, you are still unable to answer it, consider marking it and returning to it later. Not only will this reduce the time pressure that you might feel to complete the exam, but you may be presented with the same question in a different form later in the exam, which may serve to jog your memory for the correct answer. A subsequent question may also provide a definition or additional information that helps you with the answer. Additionally, by finishing the exam, those questions you skipped can be reconsidered with time pressures reduced. The afternoon session allows more time (three hours for 150 questions, or nearly a minute-and-a-half per question) and, assuming proper preparation, should prove less stressful to complete.

Most importantly, you should practice the above-mentioned principle of concentration when taking the examination. Clear your mind of extraneous thoughts; the only thing that matters is the exam question in front of you. Distractions ("Am I going to pass?" "Will I have time to catch my flight?") should be acknowledged as such, and then put out of mind. The exam is most analogous to driving long distance: you need to be simultaneously concentrating on the task at hand in the moment (the question) and aware of the distance, route, and time course (the exam as a whole). If you do this, the core exam will appear both less onerous and less pressured; the exam will flow as a series of individual questions, each of which you have given your full concentration and attention.

A FINAL WORD

To build upon the excerpt quoted earlier, studying for the board exam does involve an attempt to master an ever-growing body of knowledge, and can often be a frustrating and lonely experience. However, successfully completing a review of the core material of preventive and occupational medicine is, in the long run, greater recompense for the frustrations. I found that I was able to focus on the entire field of occupational medicine in an organized and systematic fashion, and I filled in some of the blanks in my knowledge within areas I had not sufficiently covered in the practicum. My practice in occupational medicine has benefited considerably from the broadening of my knowledge that came with review and study for this exam, and this review has helped inform my teaching with students and residents in occupational medicine. Approaching the challenges of this exam with the advice offered above will, I hope, enable you to overcome them with the same positive attitude.

SELECTED REFERENCES

Core Examination

Benenson AS. *Control of Communicable Disease Manual.* 16th ed. Washington. American Public Health Association, 1995.
Cassens BJ. *Preventive Medicine and Public Health.* 2nd ed. Baltimore. Williams & Wilkins, 1992.
Last JM, Wallace RB. *Maxcy-Rosenau-Last Public Health and Preventive Medicine.* 13th ed. Norwalk, CT. Appleton & Lange, 1992.
Morton RF, Hebel JR, McCarter RJ. *A Study Guide to Epidemiology and Biostatistics.* 4th ed. Rockville, MD. Aspen Publishing, 1996.
U. S. Preventive Services Task Force. *Guide to Clinical Preventive Services.* 2nd ed. Baltimore. Williams & Wilkins, 1996.

Occupational Medicine Specialty Examination

Felton JS. *Occupational Medical Management.* Boston. Little, Brown & Co, 1989.
LaDou, J. *Occupational Medicine.* Norwalk, CT. Appleton & Lange, 1996.
Levy BS, Wegman DH. *Occupational Health: Recognizing and Preventing Work-Related Disease.* 3rd ed. Boston. Little, Brown & Co, 1995.
McCunney RJ. *A Practical Approach to Occupational and Environmental Medicine.* 2nd ed. Boston. Little, Brown & Co, 1994.
Moser R. *Effective Management of Occupational and Environmental Health and Safety Programs.* Beverly, MA. OEM Press, 1992.
Rom W. *Environmental and Occupational Medicine.* 2nd ed. Boston. Little, Brown & Co, 1994.
Rosenstock L, Cullen MR. *Textbook of Clinical Occupational and Environmental Medicine.* Philadelphia. WB Saunders Co, 1994.
Snyder JW, Klees JE, eds. *Law and the Workplace.* Occup. Med. State-of-the-Art Reviews. Vol. 11 (1) January-March, 1996. Philadelphia. Hanley & Belfus, 1996.
Zenz C, Dickerson OB, Horvath EP. *Occupational Medicine.* 3rd ed. St. Louis. Mosby-Year Book Inc, 1994.

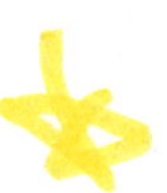

Other Useful Materials

Benson, Herbert. *The Relaxation Response.* New York. Morrow, 1975.
McNamara JJ. On taking a board examination at the age of 54. *New Engl J Med* 1995;332:1794–5
Vlachos NA, Parmet AJ, Chaulk CP. *Study Guide for Preventive Medicine Certification.* Beverly, MA. OEM Press, 1996.

Information on the *ATSDR Case Studies in Environmental Medicine* can be obtained from:
    Agency for Toxic Substances and Disease Registry
    Division of Health Education
    1600 Clifton Road, NE
    Atlanta, GA 30333

Application materials and further information on the content of the ABPM examination are available at the following address:
    American Board of Preventive Medicine, Inc.
    9950 West Lawrence Avenue
    Suite # 106
    Schiller Park, IL 60176
    847-671-1750
    WWW Homepage: http://members.aol.com/abpmnet/index.html

John D. Meyer, M.D.

Section 1

1

Occupational Medical Services

OBJECTIVES

- Discuss the scope of occupational medicine practice
- Explain the essential and elective components of such practice
- List the need for occupational medicine services
- Enumerate the various methods of delivery of occupational medicine services

OUTLINE

I. History of Occupational Medicine
II. Occupational Health Services
      Table 1–1. Occupational and environmental health programs: essential components
      Table 1–2. Elective components of occupational and environmental health programs
  A. Clinical Services
    1. Preplacement Evaluation
    2. Work-Related Injuries
        Figure 1–1. Sample medical treatment authorization form
        Figure 1–2. A sample form for reporting results of a preplacement evaluation
        Figure 1–3. A first-report form for a work-related injury
    3. Return to Work Evaluation
    4. Periodic Examinations
    5. Health Assessments
  B. Ancillary Services
  C. Nonclinical Activities
  D. Health Promotion Activities
  E. Referral Patterns
    1. Occupational Medicine Physician
    2. Local Medical Specialists
    3. Other Professionals

III. The Delivery of Occupational Medical Services
   A. Determining the Need for Occupational Medical Services
        Table 1–3. Factors in establishing the need for occupational medical services for small businesses
   B. Corporate-Sponsored Health Care Delivery
   C. Union-Sponsored Occupational Health Care
        Table 1–4. Local union health and safety involvement
   D. Hospital-Based Occupational Health Programs
   E. University-Based Teaching Centers
IV. References

KEY POINTS

- Knowledge about occupational exposure can be traced into antiquity, but it was not until the late seventeenth century that Ramazzini urged his colleagues to pay attention to diseases of the workplace. Occupational medicine has been a distinct discipline within the American Board of Preventive Medicine since 1954, but there continues to be a shortage of specialists. Most work-related problems are treated by primary care physicians.
- Over 90% of businesses in the United States and the world have 100 or fewer employees, often making it economically difficult to provide onsite health care for workers.
- Occupational health services, in their broadest sense, can include all forms of health care delivery to the working population. A variety of factors determine the types of services provided, but the American College of Occupational and Environmental Medicine (ACOEM) has published guidelines regarding essential and elective components (see Table 1–1 and Table 1–2).
- Clinical services such as preplacement and return-to-work evaluations, management of work-related injuries, periodic examinations, and other health assessments should include careful consideration of medical confidentiality. Decisions regarding work capabilities should always focus on the worker's health. Employees should be made aware of medical information reported to businesses with said information focusing on the ability to perform essential job functions.
- In the provision of occupational health services to small businesses, the following items are considered essential: an audiometric booth and audiometer with adherence to the Occupational Safety and Health Administration (OSHA) Hearing Standard, a well-functioning and calibrated spirometer with a properly trained technician, and a vision screener. It may be appropriate to include laboratory, x-ray, and physical therapy or to make provisions for these services by referral.
- The physician providing occupational health care is often viewed as a health consultant to business. Educational activities are an essential component of service delivered by the physician on such issues as the prevention and management of back injuries, substance abuse testing, and the role of lifestyle in promoting health.
- A good working professional relationship with local medical specialists such as orthopedists, general surgeons, otolaryngologists, pulmonologists, neurologists, and psychiatrists is advised. Access to professionals such as industrial hygienists, audiologists, or physical therapists can be helpful.
- The goals of an occupational health service include protecting workers from health and safety hazards, protecting the local environment, facilitating safe placement of workers, assuring adequate medical care and rehabilitation of the occupationally ill or injured, and health promotion.
- A well-run program depends on effective communication between the business facility and the physician. A visit to the business is essential. Awareness of corpo-

rate policies and union-sponsored programs can be helpful. University-based teaching centers can serve as a valuable information or referral point.

QUESTIONS

*1. Which of the following statements is **false** regarding occupational medicine and the workplace?*

A. Occupational causes of disease have been recognized since at least the eighteenth century.
B. Approximately 35% of businesses in the United States have 100 or fewer employees.
C. Occupational medicine is a new specialty in the United States, being a distinct discipline within the American Board of Preventive Medicine since 1954.
D. According to most sources, a shortage of specialists in the field of occupational medicine exists in the United States today.
E. The type of testing to be done at a preplacement examination depends on the job for which the worker is being considered.

*2. In the provision of occupational health services to small businesses, the following items are considered essential **except**:*

A. an audiometric booth and audiometer.
B. a well-functioning and calibrated spirometer.
C. a vision screener.
D. a properly trained spirometric technician.
E. a clinic-based laboratory that conducts toxicologic analysis of biologic and environmental samples.

*3. The goals of an occupational health service include the following **except**:*

A. protecting people at work from health and safety hazards.
B. assisting in measures related to personal health maintenance.
C. providing primary care for personal illness.
D. facilitating safe placement of workers according to their physical, mental, and emotional capacities.
E. assuring adequate medical care and rehabilitation of the occupationally ill and injured.

*4. According to the American College of Occupational and Environmental Medicine, all the following are considered essential components of an occupational and environmental health program **except**:*

A. medical surveillance.
B. diagnosis and treatment of occupational illnesses.
C. maintenance of occupational medical records.
D. biostatistics and epidemiology assessments.
E. immunization against nonoccupational infectious diseases.

*5. In the context of conducting a preplacement evaluation, all of the following are true **except**:*

A. The physician has no obligation to the business enterprise to report functional limitations and corresponding accommodations that may be necessary to work.

B. The physician should interpret all ancillary tests according to the employer's established criteria in order to determine if the examinee is suitable for employment.

C. The patient should be asked as to what information will be released to the employer.

D. The patient should be advised to sign an appropriate release form that allows the physician to discuss pertinent medical findings with the employer.

E. Medical advice concerning fitness for duty should be released to human resource personnel at the business.

2

Legal and Ethical Issues

OBJECTIVES

- Discuss exceptions to the exclusive remedy of workers' compensation
- Explain record-keeping requirements of OSHA and workers' compensation
- Discuss the development of workers' compensation law in our country
- List factors that determine compensability of an injury or illness
- List rules of confidentiality related to medical records of injured workers
- Identify ethical issues involved in the practice of occupational and environmental medicine
- Explain the impact of the Americans with Disabilities Act (ADA) on the workplace and occupational medicine

OUTLINE

    I. Workers' Compensation Law
      A. Determining When a Disorder is Occupational
          Table 2–1. Information provided on Material Safety Data Sheets (MSDS)
      B. Exceptions to the Exclusivity of Workers' Compensation
        1. The Intentional Tort Exception
        2. The Dual-Capacity Doctrine
      C. Obligations of the Occupational Physician
   II. Occupational Safety and Health and Other Record-Keeping and Reporting Requirements
      A. Record-Keeping Requirements
        1. OSHA Requirements
        2. Workers' Compensation Law Requirements
      B. Medical Record Access
        1. OSHA's Exposure and Medical Record Access Standard
        2. State Laws Governing Access to Medical Records
        3. Confidentiality
  III. The Americans with Disabilities Act (ADA)

KEY POINTS

- Workers' compensation statutes vary from state to state, but represent a series of compromises between employer and employee. Although generally less of a monetary recovery than through suits at common law, payment is made regardless of fault and presumably more quickly. In exchange, employees agree to accept this compensation as their exclusive remedy, based on disability and without other damages. Employees effectively give up their right to sue employers at common law with certain exceptions as outlined below. Disputes are generally decided by administrative bodies, rather than courts.

- At first, during the early development of workers' compensation, only work-related accidents were covered. Illness and disease coverage was later included if the employee's occupation put him or her at a greater risk of getting the disease than the general public or if a work-related accident aggravated or accelerated the underlying disease. Mental stress attributable to the general work environment is not covered, but cumulative trauma disorders are. As to latency of certain diseases, most states have adopted the discovery rule, with the statute of limitations beginning when the claimant becomes aware of the disease and its potential work-relatedness.

- Exceptions to the exclusivity of workers' compensation include an injury caused by a deliberate and intentional act of the employer. This might include the employer and physician if the presence of the disease was known and fraudulently concealed from the employee, resulting in an exacerbation. Furthermore, employees might be able to file cases at common law under the dual-capacity doctrine when a relationship other than an employer–employee one is established (e.g., doctor–patient). Good medical and ethical practice, as well as potential for liability, are compelling reasons for being completely candid with the employee regarding a suspected occupational disorder.

- The OSHA Hazard Communication Standard (HCS), 29 CFR 1910.1200, applicable to all employers covered by the OSHA Act (including importers of chemicals), requires that containers in the workplace be properly labeled, that employees be informed of and trained about the hazards of chemicals to which they are or may be exposed, and that Material Safety Data Sheets (MSDS) detailing the hazards of specific chemicals be made available to employees (see Table 2–1). In addition, under the Superfund Amendments and Reauthorization Act (SARA), citizens may obtain information regarding hazardous materials in their communities.

- Injuries (except extremely minor ones treated only with first aid) and all deaths and illness that result from a work-related accident or from an exposure in the work environment should be recorded on the OSHA 200 Log. This would include such conditions as skin disorders and those due to repeated trauma. Many specific requirements apply. Injuries and illnesses resulting in restricted work activity or days away from work are recordable. Employees may have access to logs where they currently or previously have worked. Accidents resulting in one or more deaths must be reported to OSHA within 48 hours. It is also imperative that physicians be familiar with the reporting requirements of the workers' compensation laws of the state in which they practice.

- OSHA's Exposure and Medical Record Access Standard "applies to all employee exposure and medical records, and analyses thereof, made or maintained in any manner, including on an in-house or contractual (fee-for-service) basis." Any employer who has employees exposed to "toxic substances" or "harmful physical agents" must provide the employee (or his or her authorized representative) access to his or her medical record within 15 days of a request. Written consent (good for up to one year) should be obtained. All medical records must be retained for the duration of the employee's employment plus 30 years. Refusal by a physician for the employer, to permit an employee direct access to his or her medical records, is allowable where the record concerns a terminal illness or a psychiatric condition and viewing it may be detrimental to the employee. However, the records must be shown to the employee's authorized representative.

- Employers are entitled to counsel about the medical fitness of individuals in relation to work, but are not entitled to diagnoses or details of a specific nature. As to work-related disorders, the employer is obliged to know about an employee's condition in order to provide protection from further exposure and to comply with necessary restrictions on that person's activities. The physician should be aware of the Code of Ethical Conduct of the ACOEM.
- Under the Americans with Disabilities Act (ADA), a disabled person is "qualified" if, with "reasonable accommodation" he or she can perform the "essential functions" of the job as well as one who is not disabled. An accommodation is necessarily reasonable if it does not impose on the employer an "undue hardship." Employment-related examinations are allowed only after an offer is made.
- Toxic tort suits are suits at common law, brought by those who claim that exposure to the toxic substance caused them some injury or disorder. Workers can sue third-party suppliers of materials to their employers (e.g., asbestos). In addition to the usual damages for medical expenses, lost earning capacity, and pain and suffering, plaintiffs who claim exposure to toxins may, in some states, seek damages for future risk of illness, fear of future illness, or the cost of medical surveillance.
- Fetal protection programs directed solely at women, solely for the protection of fetuses, are not legitimate employer policies.
- Private employer drug testing is most questionable when employers wish to test employees who do not work in safety-sensitive positions.

QUESTIONS

*1. Which of the following is **incorrect** regarding workers' compensation?*

A. Employees give up their right to sue employers at common law and agree to accept a certain sum of money per week for their inability to work as a result of work-related injuries.
B. Employees generally agree to accept this compensation as their exclusive remedy against the employer.
C. Only work-related accidents are covered, whereas work-related disease and illness are not.
D. Payment is made regardless of fault.
E. Disputes are generally decided by administrative bodies rather than courts.

*2. All of the following are true regarding the federal Hazard Communication Standard **except:***

A. If the treating physician determines that a medical emergency exists, the manufacturer must release trade secret–protected identity information.
B. Importers of chemicals are not covered.
C. Containers in the workplace that contain hazardous chemicals must be labeled with the chemical's identity, appropriate hazard warnings, and the identity of the manufacturer.
D. Employees must be trained about the hazards of chemicals to which they are or may be exposed.
E. Material Safety Data Sheets (MSDS) must be made available to employees who may be exposed to those chemicals.

3. *Information provided on Material Safety Data Sheets must include all of the following **except:***

A. the chemical names, but not the common names, of all ingredients whether they are health hazards or not.
B. the health hazards of the chemical.
C. the primary routes of exposure.
D. the OSHA permissible exposure limit.
E. whether the substance has been found to be a potential carcinogen by the International Agency for Research on Cancer or OSHA.

4. *Regarding OSHA Form 200, Log and Summary of Occupational Injuries and Illnesses:*

A. Only injuries or illnesses that result in days off work are recorded.
B. Occupational skin disorders need not be recorded.
C. A disorder due to repeated trauma or physical agents and that results in restricted work activity should be recorded.
D. Employee access to the OSHA 200 Log is limited to the logs for the establishment where the employee currently works.
E. An OSHA Form 101 must be completed for each entry in the OSHA 200 log even if the same information is reported on workers' compensation or other forms.

5. *Under OSHA's Record Access Standard, all of the following are true **except:***

A. The Standard applies to all employee exposure and medical records regardless of where they are maintained.
B. All medical records must be retained for the duration of the employee's employment plus 30 years.
C. The employee can utilize a designated representative to obtain medical record information.
D. Records regarding alcohol or drug abuse programs are considered medical records even if they are maintained apart from other medical records.
E. The employer may refuse to show medical records to the employee if the physician believes that direct access to records concerning a psychiatric condition could be detrimental.

6. *Which of the following statements is **not** true concerning legal and ethical issues in occupational medicine?*

A. According to ACOEM's Code of Ethical Conduct, employers are entitled to counsel about the medical fitness of individuals in relation to work, but are not entitled to diagnoses or details of a specific nature.
B. A disabled person is qualified if, with reasonable accommodation, he or she can perform the essential functions of the job.
C. Federally mandated drug testing applies to safety-sensitive and nonsensitive positions.
D. Toxic tort suits are suits at common law, brought by those who claim that exposure to the toxic substance caused them some injury or disorder.
E. The United States Supreme Court has found fetal protection programs directed solely at women to be unlawfully discriminatory.

3

The Role of Regulatory Agencies

OBJECTIVES

- Identify the mandates for various government agencies involved in occupational and environmental health
- List the various types of OSHA standards that impact on the practice of occupational medicine

OUTLINE

Table 3–1. Federal agencies with rules that affect the practice of occupational and environmental medicine

I. The Occupational Safety and Health Administration
  A. Occupational Injuries and Illnesses
  Table 3–2. OSHA standards that impact occupational medicine
  Table 3–3. OSHA chemical specific standards
  B. Access to Employee Medical Records
  C. Occupational Noise Exposure
  D. Physical Fitness Evaluations
  E. Medical Services and First Aid
  F. Chemical Specific Standards
  G. Blood-Borne Pathogens
  H. Hazard Communication
  I. Occupational Exposure to Hazardous Chemicals in Laboratories
II. National Institute for Occupational Safety and Health
  A. Health Hazard Evaluations
  B. Training and Publications
III. Mine Safety and Health Administration
IV. Nuclear Regulatory Commission
 V. Department of Transportation
  A. Federal Aviation Administration
  B. Federal Railroad Administration
  C. Federal Highway Administration

KEY POINTS

- OSHA standards, National Institute for Occupational Safety and Health (NIOSH) research activities, and certain Environmental Protection Agency (EPA) regulations should become familiar topics for physicians who provide occupational health care.
- OSHA standards apply to recordability of occupational injuries and illnesses, access to employee medical records, occupational noise exposure, medical services and first aid, exposure to blood-borne pathogens, hazard communication, required medical surveillance for specific operations and chemicals, and a number of other areas. However, OSHA does not cover federal, state, or local municipal employers. State OSHA standards are often identical to federal OSHA standards and in some cases, may be more stringent. Compliance with employee requests for medical records is required within 15 working days.
- Recordability of a condition as an injury as opposed to an illness depends on the duration of exposure. An injury results from an instantaneous exposure. Recordability of occupational injuries is in part determined by the requirement for medical treatment as opposed to first-aid care (where simple treatment with over-the-counter medication may be required). First-aid care for injuries is not recordable.
- The OSHA standard for occupational noise exposure requires annual examinations for employees exposed to noise of 85 dB or higher on a daily time-weighted average (TWA) basis. Audiograms that show a standard threshold shift (STS) of 10 dB or greater compared with baseline must be evaluated by an audiologist or physician to determine the need for further evaluation. A work-related change in hearing of 25 dB averaged over the frequencies of 2,000, 3,000, and 4,000 Hz is recordable on the OSHA 200 Log.
- Several OSHA standards require the employee to have a medical examination to determine physical fitness to perform certain jobs, or to wear specific personal protective equipment (e.g., respirators). However, not all of these standards specify the content of these medical examinations or their frequency (e.g., respirator standard). There are detailed individual standards for 26 chemicals, each of which includes a section on medical surveillance. Medical surveillance is typically required when airborne exposure levels exceed 50% of the permissible exposure limit (PEL) for at least 30 days per year. Certain of these standards have provisions for medical removal from work (such as the lead standard for general industry).
- After completion of the medical surveillance examination, the physician must furnish a written opinion regarding risk as well as fitness for or limitations in use of personal protective equipment.
- NIOSH is a part of the Centers for Disease Control (CDC), and protects the health and safety of workers by conducting research on workplace hazards, providing information pertinent to the development of OSHA standards through criteria documents and current intelligence bulletins (CIBs), and conducting health hazard evaluations (HHEs) at the request of employees or employers. NIOSH also provides training through Educational Resource Centers (ERCs) for occupational medicine residents and graduate students in occupational nursing, industrial hygiene, and safety.
- The EPA is responsible for implementation of numerous acts of Congress promulgated to protect the environment. While it is not necessary for most occupational physicians to have detailed knowledge of the specifics of environmental laws and regulations promulgated by bodies like the EPA, it is desirable for them to become

more knowledgeable concerning the concepts and process of risk assessment. The Toxic Substance Control Act (TSCA) requires manufacturers or users of a specific chemical to keep a record of any allegation of a heretofore unknown adverse health effect, and to report to the EPA new information that reasonably supports the conclusion that the chemical or mixture presents a substantial risk of injury to health or the environment. The Agency for Toxic Substances and Disease Registry (ATSDR) provides continuing education training for physicians through case studies in environmental medicine.

- Other agencies may impact the practice of the occupational medicine physician such as the Mine Safety and Health Administration (MSHA). The purpose of this agency is similar to that of OSHA except it covers only workers in the mining industry. The Nuclear Regulatory Commission (NRC) has primary responsibility for regulating hazards from ionizing radiation, including x-rays, gamma rays, and radioactive material that can be taken into the body. Agencies of the Department of Transportation (DOT), such as the Federal Aviation Administration (FAA), Federal Railroad Administration, and the Federal Highway Administration (FHA) set physical qualification standards for their employees and issue regulations dealing with drug and alcohol testing. The Equal Employment Opportunity Commission (EEOC) is charged with enforcing the Americans with Disabilities Act.

QUESTIONS

*1. Which of the following statements regarding the Occupational Safety and Health Administration (OSHA) is **incorrect**?*

A. The Occupational Safety and Health (OSH) Act does not cover federal, state, or local municipal employees.
B. OSHA standard requires annual examinations for employees exposed to noise of 80 dB or higher on a daily time-weighted average (TWA) basis.
C. After completion of a required medical surveillance examination under OSHA, the physician must furnish a written opinion that includes any limitations on the use of personal protective equipment.
D. The OSHA standard for lead in general industry (29 CFR 1910.1025) has provisions for medical removal protection based on monitoring of whole blood lead levels.
E. Each of OSHA's chemical specific standards includes a section on medical surveillance.

2. Under OSHA record keeping requirements:

A. Only certain work-related illnesses are recordable.
B. An injury that requires first aid is recordable.
C. Over-the-counter medication is considered first aid and is, therefore, recordable.
D. Compliance with employee requests for medical records is required within 15 working days.
E. All standard threshold shifts noted on annual audiometry are recordable.

*3. All of the following chemicals have a specific OSHA standard **except:***

A. asbestos
B. 1,1,2-trichloroethylene
C. formaldehyde
D. vinyl chloride
E. benzene

4. *All of the following statements regarding OSHA standards are true **except:***

A. Federal OSHA standards must be more stringent than state OSHA standards.
B. OSHA's definition of an injury is something that is caused by an instantaneous exposure.
C. The OSHA Blood-Borne Pathogen Standard (29 CFR 1910.1030) is directed primarily at the health care industry.
D. The Hazardous Waste Operations and Emergency Response Standard (29 CFR 1910.120) requires the employee to have a medical examination to determine physical fitness.
E. The Respiratory Protection Standard (29 CFR 1910.134) does not specify details of the content of the medical examination.

5. *The National Institute for Occupational Safety and Health (NIOSH):*

A. has responsibility for enforcing OSHA regulations.
B. is part of the Department of Labor.
C. is not allowed to conduct research.
D. may conduct Health Hazard Evaluations (HHEs) at the request of employers.
E. accredits residency training programs in occupational medicine.

6. *Which of the following is true concerning roles or requirements of various agencies?*

A. NIOSH develops health standards for OSHA.
B. OSHA requires that a physician determine a worker's ability to wear a respirator every 12 months.
C. The Equal Employment Opportunity Commission (EEOC) is charged with enforcing the Americans with Disabilities Act (ADA).
D. The Agency for Toxic Substances and Disease Registry (ATSDR) is responsible for regulating imported chemicals.
E. Under the Toxic Substance Control Act (TSCA), physicians are required to report adverse effects of chemicals to the Agency for Toxic Substances and Disease Registry (ATSDR).

REFERENCES

Doyle JR. Access to medical record standard. *Occup. Env. Med. Rep.* 3:53, 1989.

The Establishment of an Occupational Health Program

OBJECTIVES

- Identify steps necessary for the development of an occupational health program
- Illustrate types of primary prevention programs for the work site
- Identify examples of secondary prevention programs in occupational medicine
- List issues involved in clinical management of work-related injury or illness
- Illustrate the benefits of the walk-through visit at the work site and review the components of that evaluation

OUTLINE

    I. Assessment
            Table 4–1. Guidelines for the physician conducting a facility walk-
            through
   II. Development and Operation
        A. Primary Prevention Programs
            1. Properly Designed Workplace
            2. Matching Workers to the Job
                Figure 4–1. Elemental job analysis
            3. Worker Training
            4. Industrial Hygiene
        B. Secondary Prevention Programs
            1. Medical Surveillance
            2. Employee Assistance Program
        C. Tertiary Prevention Programs
            1. On-Site Services
            2. Team Management of Cases
            3. Case Management
  III. The Walk-Through Survey
        A. Initial Recognition of Hazards

B. The Systematic Approach to a Walk-Through Survey
C. Relationship with Industrial Hygienists
IV. References

KEY POINTS

- An understanding of the activities of the organization is critical to the development of a quality occupational health program. The initial assessment includes conducting a walk-through of the facility (see Table 4–1).
- The delivery of occupational medical care has expanded from the industrial in-plant clinic to hospital-based clinics, multispecialty groups, and occupational medicine programs within academic settings. These settings should identify a contact person both at the business and at the clinic to enhance communication regarding occupational and medical services.
- Prevention has three components: primary, secondary, and tertiary.
- Primary prevention is an intervention that addresses a risk factor for a disease or injury. Key approaches to primary prevention include a properly designed and ergonomically sound workplace, matching workers to the job through functional job descriptions, regular training (the majority of injuries occur in recently hired people), and industrial hygiene.
- Industrial hygiene involves the recognition, evaluation, and control of industrial hazards that may cause illness among workers. Industrial hazards frequently encountered by workers include chemicals, physical energy (such as electromagnetic and ionizing radiation), noise, vibration, repetitive motion, temperature extremes, and microorganisms. In addition to routine industrial hygiene assessments, other situations requiring evaluation include development of a new process, change in a process, or situations in which air levels of chemicals are above specified thresholds.
- Secondary prevention refers to early detection of disease and intervention before symptoms appear. The goal is to reverse, halt, or retard the progression of a disorder. Key approaches include medical surveillance (with biologic monitoring as appropriate), early identification of repetitive motion disorders and high-risk manual-lifting situations, elimination of various physical hazards, and development of employee assistance programs. Biologic monitoring is an attempt to assess the internal dose of overall worker exposure to chemicals in the workplace through measurement of the appropriate determinant in biologic specimens such as urine, blood, or exhaled air. Biologic monitoring has advantages over air monitoring.
- Tertiary prevention refers to minimizing the effects of disease and disability by reducing complications and premature deterioration and assuring a timely return to work.
- Maintaining an on-site program can be a cost-effective method of delivering occupational health services for many organizations, depending on the number of employees and the complexity and health risks of the operations. Occupational health nurses and physicians as well as physical therapists and other allied health professionals can enhance the delivery of administrative and clinical occupational health functions on site. Injured employees who do not use the plant medical facilities may require case management.
- Where feasible, the physician should review plant operations through a walk-through survey and with an industrial hygienist, who can comment on the hazards present and the adequacy of the respective control measures to protect workers from those hazards. The recognition of these hazards should include assessment of physical factors as outlined above, as well as the three primary routes of exposure to chemical agents (inhalation, ingestion, and skin contact). Transplacental absorption may be a consideration in women of childbearing age. Determinants of absorption such as the physical form of the agent, chemical characteristics, particle size and dimension, and hygiene practices are also important factors.

QUESTIONS

1. *Which of the following questions is **least** important to the occupational physician conducting a facility walk-through?*

A. Are there substances used in the workplace for which established OSHA standards exist?
B. What is the human resource policy regarding utilization of a sick leave?
C. What staff members are responsible for health and safety measures?
D. Are modified duty assignments available?
E. What types of personal protective equipment are used?

2. *Which of the following statements is **incorrect** regarding the three levels of prevention?*

A. Primary prevention is any intervention that addresses a risk factor for a disease or injury.
B. Screening mammography is a type of primary prevention.
C. Periodic cytologic testing of the uterine cervix (Papanicolaou smear) is a form of secondary prevention.
D. Biologic monitoring of construction workers for lead is an example of secondary prevention.
E. The care of pressure sores in bedridden patients is a form of tertiary prevention.

3. *Biologic monitoring of the worker has advantage over air monitoring of the work environment because:*

A. biologic monitoring takes into account absorption via routes other than inhalation.
B. environmental measurements rarely correlate with adverse health effects.
C. biologic monitoring is not substantially altered by the insignificant contributions of personal hygiene habits during activities such as eating and smoking in the work environment.
D. biologic monitoring results will not vary with the respiratory rate of the individual worker.
E. environmental monitoring is almost never feasible.

4. *Which of the following is most true concerning the provision of on-site occupational health services to industry?*

A. Maintaining an on-site program is never cost-effective, but is preferred by businesses because employees desire it.
B. Only administrative activities and not clinical activities should be conducted in such settings.
C. Due to conflict of interests, the on-site medical facility should not be located within the work site, but rather directly next door to the plant.
D. Space for an on-site program is not usually an important consideration.
E. On-site services can be enhanced by the availability of a physical therapist.

5. *Which of the following routes of exposure **is least** relevant to the occupational setting?*

A. inhalation
B. transplacental
C. ingestion
D. dermatologic
E. parenteral

6. When considering exposure by inhalation:

A.   only the alveoli are subject to injury.

B.   the largest particles and aerosols exceeding 10 μm in diameter usually deposit throughout the bronchiole system.

C.   fibers that are less than 5 μm in diameter may deposit throughout the respiratory tract.

D.   hazardous agents may be absorbed directly into the systemic circulation unlike the skin where the effects are always local.

E.   gases and vapors tend to irritate the alveoli predominantly because they always reach the deep lung tissue.

REFERENCES

Documentation of the threshold limit values and biological exposure indices, 7th ed. Cincinnati: American College of Industrial Hygienists, 1991.

Hatch TF, Gross P. *Pulmonary deposition and retention of aerosols.* New York: Academic, 1964.

5

The Americans with Disabilities Act

OBJECTIVES

- Explain the relationship between impairment and disability
- Discuss the basic provisions of the Americans with Disabilities Act (ADA)
- Explain the impact of this law on the practice of occupational medicine
- List the types of examinations allowed by employers under the ADA
- Explain the process involved in determination of fitness for duty

OUTLINE

IV. ADA Information Flow
>   Figure 5–4. Report of preplacement medical examination
V. ADA's Impact: Two Views
>   A. ADA: A Costly Burden
>   B. ADA: A Beneficial Opportunity
VI. References

KEY POINTS

- The ADA was built on many provisions of sections 503 and 504 of the Rehabilitation Act of 1973, which covered government employees and federal contractors. The Civil Rights Act of 1991 strengthened the ADA by allowing punitive and compensatory damages. There are several definitions related to the ADA legislation (see Table 5–1).
- The ADA places strong emphasis on evaluation of each individual situation on a case-by-case basis. The relationship between impairment, functional limitation, and disability varies enormously from individual to individual. Disability determination is a nonmedical managerial task, whereas health professionals make medical technical judgments about pathology, impairment, and functional limitation within a framework of generally accepted medical principles and practice. The ADA places clear responsibility on management to make appropriate decisions about disability, direct threat, and reasonable accommodation.
- The ADA prohibits preoffer, preemployment medical inquiries, medical examinations, and other medical information gathering (e.g., workers' compensation claims) until after a bona fide job offer has been made. Job application forms may ask only about current ability to perform essential job functions. The job offer may be conditioned on satisfactory completion of a postoffer medical examination as long as this is required of all other entering employees in the same job category. Strength testing and agility tests are not considered to be medical procedures, and may be required preoffer. Withdrawal of a job offer must be job-related (to essential functions) and consistent with business necessity, not based on speculation of future injury, and may occur only if reasonable accommodation is not possible or poses an undue hardship for the employer.
- For current employees, medical surveillance and fitness-for-duty examinations can be required only when mandated by statute or when job related and consistent with business necessity, and then they must be limited to determining ability to perform essential functions on a case-by-case basis. Note: most often, OSHA standards require the employer to offer examinations, but they do not have to be taken. An exception is audiometry under the hearing conservation standard.
- Voluntary examinations (e.g., blood pressure, cholesterol screening, health risk appraisal, periodic physician exam, wellness programs) are permitted.
- The ADA requires that confidential medical records be maintained by the employer in locked cabinets, separate from personnel files, accessible only to designated persons. The applicant/employee should sign a medical release authorizing dissemination of medical information. The ADA requires that health professionals share sufficient information with employers to make management decisions about the presence of a disability, direct threat, and reasonable accommodation.
- The medical examiner should not be lured into making employment decisions or determining whether a reasonable accommodation can be made. He/she should advise the employer about two things only: (1) the individual's functional abilities and limitations in relation to functional job requirements, and (2) whether the individual can perform the job without posing a direct threat to the health or safety of him/herself or others. The ADA does not permit blanket exclusions.
- Testing for illegal drugs is specifically excluded as being a "medical test." The Equal Employment Opportunity Commission (EEOC) has recommended informally that

employers arrange drug testing so that any associated medical inquiry is conducted after a conditional job offer. The ADA offers limited protection to recovered/recovering alcoholics and illegal drug users. The critical distinction for illegal drug users is between current and former use. Employers are not required to provide alcohol/drug rehabilitation as a reasonable accommodation.

* The ADA's definition of "any mental or psychological disorder" is very broad. Nowhere else were symptoms or diagnoses included or excluded with the same degree of specificity (e.g., of exclusions: pyromania, homosexuality, pedophilia). Stress and depression may or may not be considered impairments, depending on whether these conditions result from a documented psychological or mental disorder. Functional job descriptions can include a number of attributes in the psychological and social realm (e.g., maintain concentration over time).

QUESTIONS

*1. Key terms used in the ADA include all of the following **except:***

A. direct threat.
B. preexisting condition.
C. reasonable accommodation.
D. bona fide job offer.
E. essential job functions.

*2. Which of the following would **not** be considered as a disability under the ADA?*

A. A physical or mental impairment that substantially limits one or more of the major life activities
B. A record of having such an impairment
C. Being regarded as having an impairment
D. Being blind
E. Current use of illegal drugs

*3. Reasonable accommodation as defined by the ADA may include any of the following **except:***

A. changes to a job application process.
B. modification of the work environment or job structure.
C. equal benefits and privileges.
D. opportunity to perform essential job functions.
E. a requirement that the employee pay for assistive equipment.

*4. Factors to be considered in evaluating a direct threat to oneself or others include all **but** which one of the following:*

A. ability to perform essential job functions.
B. imminence of potential harm.
C. nature and severity of potential harm.
D. likelihood that potential harm will occur.
E. duration of risk.

5. Under the ADA, current employees may be subject to which of the following:

A. all tests but drug tests.
B. all tests but drug and alcohol tests.
C. all tests except for those related to workers' compensation injuries.
D. only tests that relate to essential job functions.

E. drug tests and those relating to essential job functions.

6. *Under the ADA, fitness for duty must be determined in accordance with which method?*

A. Equal Employment Opportunity Commission Medical Guidelines
B. Medical standards in the AMA Guides to the Evaluation of Permanent Impairment
C. Taking into consideration the nature of the individual disability and the nature of the job on an individual basis
D. Professionally approved practice guidelines
E. Employer's approved job qualification standards

7. *Under the ADA, preplacement medical examinations may be conducted only when:*

A. the medical examiner has been given a list of essential job functions.
B. all applicants for a particular job receive identical examinations.
C. a negative urine drug test has been reported.
D. a job offer has been made.
E. current employees are first offered newly available jobs.

8. *Which of the following statements concerning the confidentiality of medical records is inconsistent with the provisions of the ADA?*

A. Confidential medical records should be maintained by the employer in locked cabinets, separate from personnel files.
B. Records should be accessible only to designated persons.
C. Supervisors should have a record of the names of all medications taken by an employee in the event of an emergency.
D. Health professionals should share sufficient information with employers to allow them to make management decisions about reasonable accommodation.
E. The applicant/employee should sign a medical release authorizing dissemination of medical information.

6

The Role of the Occupational Health Nurse

OBJECTIVE

- List the roles of the occupational health nurse in the contemporary work site

OUTLINE

    I. Historical Perspectives
   II. Role of the Occupational Health Nurse
 III. Scope of Occupational Health Nursing
       Table 6–1. Examples of occupational health nursing practice activities within a prevention framework
 IV. Conclusion
  V. References

KEY POINTS

- Occupational health nursing is the application of principles to conserve the health of workers in all occupations. It emphasizes prevention, recognition, and treatment of illnesses and injuries, with appropriate development of nursing diagnoses and a plan of care. It requires special skills and knowledge in the fields of health education and counseling, environmental health, rehabilitation, and human relations. Occupational health nursing is a part of a multidisciplinary team approach.
- Five major functional roles of the occupational health nurse have been identified: clinician, administrator, educator, researcher, and consultant. As clinician, the nurse applies the steps of the traditional nursing process (i.e., assessment, diagnosis, planning, implementation, and evaluation). The administrator determines the resource needs of the occupational health unit and collaborates with others in its smooth management. As educator, the nurse assesses the needs of the work force with respect to health information and educational interventions for individual patients as well as groups. The occupational health nurse researcher may focus on identifying trends in

illness and injury that may stimulate a research investigation. Finally, the nurse consultant serves as a resource to management and members of the occupational health and safety team.

- External and internal factors to the organization that play a major role in the type and methods of nursing care delivered include economic constraints and resource allocation, demographics and size of the work-force population, applicable legislation, advances in technology, corporate culture concerning workplace health and hazards, and interdisciplinary team resources.
- The occupational health nurse contributes at all levels of prevention, including an emphasis on cost containment that preserves and improves quality health services (see Table 6–1). Scope of activities include health hazard assessment and surveillance, primary health care and counseling, health promotion/protection, administration, management, quality assurance, research, community orientation (development of a network of resources within the community).
- The occupational health nurse must be familiar with the laws that govern the occupational safety and health of workers (e.g., OSHA, ADA) as well as those relevant to nursing practice, proper physician supervision, and confidentiality. The Code of Ethics of the American Association of Occupational Health Nurses provides guidance for ethical decision making and addresses provision of nondiscriminatory health care, collaboration with other health professionals/agencies, confidentiality, provision of quality care, accountability, competence, and participation in knowledge-building activities such as research.

QUESTIONS

*1. The Code of Ethics of the American Association of Occupational Health Nurses provides guidance for ethical decision making and addresses all of the following areas **except:***

A. provision of nondiscriminatory health care in the work environment with regard for human dignity.
B. specification of a minimum number of continuing nursing education credits.
C. collaboration with other health professionals/agencies to meet the needs of the work force.
D. protection of the employee's right to privacy and protection of confidential information.
E. maintenance of individual competence.

2. The primary emphasis in occupational health nursing is:

A. providing primary care to workers.
B. providing for the maintenance, improvement, and protection of worker health.
C. keeping accurate OSHA logs.
D. conducting workplace inspections and surveillance.
E. investigating illness and injury trends.

3. As a direct care provider, a component of the occupational health nurse's role is to:

A. develop a nursing diagnosis and plan of care regarding the worker health problem/condition.
B. assess the health education needs of the work force.
C. conduct quality assurance activities.
D. provide advice about occupational health services to management.
E. all of the above.

4. *A major aspect of community orientation in occupational health nursing practice*
   is to:

A. provide community health fairs.
B. obtain community financial support.
C. develop a network of resources for occupational health programming.
D. identify community health specialists.
E. become politically astute.

5. *Which of the following functions is least consistent with the duties of an*
   occupational health services administrator?

A. Assessing the health information needs of the work force
B. Developing policies and procedures for all areas of the company
C. Administering influenza vaccine
D. Determining human and operational resources for the occupational health unit
E. Supervising employee assistance providers

6. *Work hardening is an example of:*

A. primary prevention.
B. secondary prevention.
C. tertiary prevention.
D. primary care.
E. physical therapy.

REFERENCES

American Association of Occupational Health Nurses. *A guide to establishing a comprehensive occupational health service.* Atlanta: AAOHN, 1987.

7

The Disability/Impairment Evaluation

OBJECTIVES

- State the purposes and components of the independent medical evaluation
- Discuss issues concerning injury or illness causality
- Identify the differences between impairment and disability
- Delineate the uses of the functional performance assessment

OUTLINE

KEY POINTS

- Independent Medical Evaluations (IMEs) are examinations performed by a physician not involved in the person's care for the purpose of clarifying medical and job issues. Key issues associated with an IME differ from clinical consultations in role and focus.
- IMEs are performed to provide information for case management and for evidence in hearings and other legal proceedings.
- IMEs are a component of all workers' compensation statutes, although the specifics vary by state. The physician must be impartial and unbiased in performing the assessment. Key issues in an IME include diagnoses, causal relationship, prognosis, maximum medical improvement, permanent impairment, work capacity, disability, appropriateness of care, and recommendations. The examinee is not necessarily a willing participant. Physicians with some clinical, consulting, or teaching involvement are considered to be more credible than those who perform only IMEs.
- Pain, especially chronic pain, may not be associated with significant physical pathology. Pathology may be present without symptoms or dysfunction. Impairment is a measurable decrement in some physiologic function, whereas disability considers not only the physical or mental impairment but also the social, psychological, or vocational factors associated with a person's ability to work. Functional limitations are manifestations of impairment.
- Work-related causation is defined as a problem that "arose out of and during the course of employment." Establishing causation to a reasonable degree of medical probability implies that it is more probable than not (i.e., there is more than a 50% probability) that a certain condition arose out of or in the course of work duties. Possibility implies less than 50% likelihood. Apportionment refers to the extent to which a problem is caused by various factors. Aggravation implies a long-standing effect due to an event, resulting in a worsening, hastening, or deterioration of the condition. Exacerbation is a temporary increase in symptoms from the condition.
- Impairment is the loss of, the loss of use of, or a derangement of any body part, system, or function. Disability is the limiting loss of the capacity to meet personal, social, or occupational demands, or to meet statutory or regulatory requirements. Impairment is a measurable decrement in health status evaluated by medical means. Maximal medical improvement is a phrase used to indicate when further recovery and restoration of function can no longer be anticipated to a reasonable degree of medical probability and implies that a condition is permanent and static. The medical role usually is limited to evaluating impairment, not disability. An impairment evaluation is based on activities of daily living and not specific tasks of employment. For most organ systems, the impairment rating guidance is broad. For example, with the skin, each category of impairment spreads across 10 percentage points. Impairment ratings were never intended to be the major factor in determining compensation for permanent impairment. Pain is usually considered in determining impairment only if substantiated by objective findings affecting both organic systems and function.
- Functional performance assessments are more accurate determinations of ability, if the assessment is valid and reliable and relates to particular jobs. Various methodologies are available. It is customary to express work capacity following parameters in the *Dictionary of Occupational Titles,* U.S. Department of Labor. Estimates of lifting and carrying capabilities are usually noted for specific frequencies. Guidelines should be provided for the frequency and duration of tasks such as bending, squatting, etc.
- In conducting an evaluation and preparing a report, it is important to review the medical records before the evaluation and to read correspondence from the client, so that the evaluation can be structured to answer specific questions. Histories need to be comprehensive, including preexisting status, specifics of injury, clinical his-

tory, and current status. Pain inventories may be helpful in identifying behavioral and psychological components related to an illness or injury. The relationship between subjective complaints and objective findings should be discussed. Available diagnostic studies should be reviewed. Additional studies may be recommended to the referring source; however, they should not be obtained without approval from the referral source to avoid conflicts regarding fiscal responsibilities for the testing. At the beginning of the visit, the physician should explain the nature of the evaluation and that an independent evaluation will be conducted, but that no treatment will be performed. There is no patient–physician relationship, and a report will be sent to the requesting client. A signed release to this effect is advised.

QUESTIONS

1. All of the following statements are true of independent medical evaluations
   except:

A. Examinations are also referred to as impartial or neutral evaluations, or agreed examinations.
B. They differ from clinical consultations in role and focus.
C. Their primary focus is to provide information for case management and evidence in hearing and other legal proceedings.
D. The evaluating physician is often involved in a treating capacity with the examinee.
E. They are a component of all workers' compensation statutes.

2. Evaluations of work-related injury require an understanding of several concepts. All of the following are true ***except:***

A. Chronic pain is usually associated with significant physical pathology.
B. Pathology may be present without symptoms or dysfunction.
C. Impairment is a measurable decrement in physiologic functioning.
D. Functional limitations are manifestations of impairment.
E. Disability relates to inability to perform activities of daily living and/or ability to work.

3. Causation is a critical issue in workers' compensation. All the following statements are true ***except:***

A. A work-related problem is one that "arose out of and during the course of employment."
B. "A reasonable degree of medical probability" refers to an event being more probable than not.
C. A certainty of at least 95% is required to establish probable cause.
D. States may vary in definitions of causation, particularly for cumulative trauma disorders, psychiatric conditions, and preexisting conditions.
E. Apportionment refers to the extent to which a problem is caused by various factors.

4. Maximum medical improvement:

A. occurs when further recovery and restoration of function can no longer be anticipated to a reasonable degree of medical probability.
B. is not a medical determination.
C. is not equivalent to the term *permanent and static.*
D. is not required to perform a permanent impairment evaluation.
E. is usually defined by set time frames rather than clinical assessment.

5. *All the following are true about permanent impairment **except** that impairment is:*

A. the loss of, loss of use of, or derangement of any body part, system, or function.
B. a measurable decrement in health status evaluated by medical means.
C. indicative of a person's ability or inability to do tasks or a set of tasks relating to work.
D. actually based on activities of daily living.
E. not synonymous with disability.

6. *All of the following are true about performing independent medical evaluations **except:***

A. Histories need to be comprehensive, including preexisting status, specifics of injury, clinical history, and current status.
B. Pain inventories, including pain drawings, may be performed as part of the assessment.
C. Radiographic studies should be obtained routinely at the time of the evaluation for the region involved.
D. Treatment is not performed as part of an independent evaluation.
E. The results of the evaluation are typically sent to the requesting client and not the examinee.

7. *Regarding functional performance assessments, all of the following are true **except:***

A. They are more accurate determinations of ability if the assessment is valid and reliable and relates to a particular job.
B. There is only one accepted methodology currently available in the United States.
C. It is customary to express work capacity following parameters in the *Dictionary of Occupational Titles,* U.S. Department of Labor, which are based primarily on lifting requirements.
D. Estimates of lifting and carrying capabilities are noted for specific frequencies.
E. Guidelines should be provided for the frequency and duration of tasks such as bending, crouching, squatting, pushing/pulling, climbing stairs, climbing ladders, reaching above shoulder level, lifting above shoulder level, balancing, and working on uneven ground or at heights.

REFERENCES

Babitsky S, Sewall HD. *Understanding the AMA Guides in workers' compensation.* Colorado Springs: Wiley Law Publications, 1992.
Larson A. *The law of workmen's compensation.* New York: Matthew Bender, 1982.
Loesser JD. What is chronic pain? *Theor. Med.* 12:213, 1991.
Ryley JF, Ahern DK, Follick MJ. Chronic pain and functional impairment: assessing beliefs about their relationship. *Arch. Phys. Med. Rehab.* 69:579, 1988.
Spektor S. Chronic pain and pain-related disabilities. *J. Disabil.* 1:98, 1990.
Tompkins N. Independent medical examinations: the how, when, and why of this useful process. *OSHA Compl. Adv.* 215:7, 1992.
Vasudevan SV. The relationship between pain and disability: an overview of the problem. *J. Disabil.* 2:44, 1991.
Vasudevan SV. Impairment, disability, and functional capacity assessment. In: Turk DC, Melzack R, eds. *Handbook of pain assessment.* New York: Guilford Press, 1992.

8

Working with the Business Community

OBJECTIVE

- Explain the influence of changing government regulation on the practice of occupational medicine

OUTLINE

KEY POINTS

- In contrast to the decline of corporate-sponsored services, there has been a substantial increase in interest in the provision of occupational health services to small businesses. Close associations with employers are becoming a paramount positioning strategy for both physicians and medical centers as the private sector assumes greater influence in health care funding and medical service delivery. Health care delivery is moving toward managed competition, with greater emphasis on employer responsibility and provider recognition of occupational health as a prudent diversification strategy. The deregulatory fervor of the 1980s has been overshadowed by public health regulation, as evidenced by such recent initiatives as the Americans with Disabilities Act, the Drug-Free Workplace Act, and the OSHA Blood-Borne

Pathogens Standard. Environmental health issues will attract more attention of business and medicine and demand additional expertise of health care providers.

- The changing occupational health environment involves providing assistance to employers, especially smaller ones, on regulatory, policy, and medical areas. Health care cost control is a major motivator for employers to establish partnerships with providers. Reimbursement for workers' compensation-related medical care is becoming more tightly controlled through the use of nurse managers and other "gatekeepers." Workers' compensation reform will ultimately force both providers and employers to become more prevention oriented.
- The successful occupational physician of the 1990s will be adept at organizational dynamics, consumer education, entrepreneurship, and marketing, along with the clinical practice of medicine. Physicians will be evaluated on both their ability to address broad community health care concerns and their clinical skills. Accordingly, prevention is likely to assume a more pronounced role, both in reducing workplace risk factors and in using the workplace as a forum for health education. The occupational medicine physician must work as part of a team, deal with multiple constituencies, show leadership, and appreciate the pressures under which organizations operate without compromising patient care or ethical principles. Partnering with hospitals can be a competitive tool.
- A board-certified occupational physician can work in academia, government, or private industry as well as in traditional settings, such as medical offices and hospitals.
- A hospital-based program provides several competitive advantages: one-stop shopping, financial resources to withstand a development period that may last 12 to 18 months, management/finance/marketing, and life support services. Unlike the past, where injury care and other occupational health-related services were loosely provided out of hospital emergency departments, today, injury care is bundled with other health-related services to create a defined product line. Physicians in hospital-based programs are able to negotiate a variety of compensation packages.
- The freestanding occupational health clinic is likely to provide the physician with greater autonomy; it also gives employers an impression of greater efficiency, easier access, and less cost than services provided by hospitals. The size of clinics varies. Offering occupational medicine services may increase patient base in a primary care practice. The era of the freestanding injury mill is ending.
- As a consultant, the more compelling opportunity may be to develop a relatively narrow niche of expertise and provide replicable services to large numbers of organizations. Examples include advice related to medical surveillance, training, health policy, program development, regulatory compliance, workers' compensation loss control, and managed care.
- The physician can (1) gain a basic foundation in occupational medicine, (2) address the range of occupational medicine, (3) remain abreast of regulatory measures, (4) address interventions in terms of health care cost containment, (5) be an educator, (6) be prepared to play multiple roles, and (7) commit to professional and aggressive marketing.
- In the future, the relationship between employer and provider will address two central issues: cost control and continually improved productivity to maintain a competitive edge in an increasingly global economy.

QUESTIONS

*1. All of the following are indicative of the changing occupational medicine environment **except:***

A. Opportunities to work with the business community are limited in the 1990s.
B. The deregulatory fervor of the 1980s has diminished and is being replaced by an emphasis on public health regulation.

  C. A profound change in occupational medicine involves a shift from fee-for-service to managed care arrangements.

  D. Health care cost control leads the agenda for many employers who recognize that partnerships with providers, especially physicians, are an essential ingredient for addressing complex occupational health issues.

  E. Employers are rapidly becoming the leading gatekeepers of the nation's health care system.

2. *Which of the following is **least** representative of the changing physician role in occupational medicine?*

  A. Physicians are not evaluated on clinical expertise but on their ability to address broader community health care concerns.

  B. Prevention is likely to assume a more pronounced role, both in reducing workplace exposures and in using the workplace as a forum for health education.

  C. The successful physician of the 1990s will be as adept at organizational dynamics, consumer education, entrepreneurship, and marketing as with the clinical practice of medicine.

  D. The occupational medicine physician is well advised to maintain as much independence as possible in order to retain flexibility in an ever-increasing market.

  E. A strong occupational medicine physician should possess the ability to work with multiple constituencies.

3. *Which of the following best characterizes hospital-based occupational health programs?*

  A. Hospital-based occupational health programs are increasingly located in emergency departments.

  B. Injury care treatment and management should function as the core of a hospital-based occupational health program.

  C. Hospitals possess the financial backing, breadth of services, and management support to prosper in competitive markets.

  D. Compensation for medical directors of hospital-based programs is usually straight salary.

  E. A hospital setting is especially attractive for the physician who prefers autonomy and independence.

4. *Which of the following does **not** characterize the opportunities inherent in a freestanding occupational health program?*

  A. Many successful clinics are large and multispecialty, while others may involve only a few physicians or a single practitioner.

  B. A freestanding occupational health clinic is likely to provide the physician with greater autonomy and gives employers an impression of greater efficiency, easier access, and less cost than services provided by hospitals.

  C. Many primary care physicians have sought to increase their patient base by offering occupational medicine services as an adjunct to an existing primary care practice.

  D. As a result of lower overhead, freestanding occupational medicine clinics tend to be more profitable than other delivery options.

  E. The era of the freestanding clinic with a dedicated focus to injury care management is beginning to slip away.

5. *Which of the following are **not** cited as compelling consultative opportunities for a physician specialist in occupational medicine?*

A. medical surveillance
B. worker-management mediation
C. worker education
D. health and safety policy and program development
E. workers' compensation loss control and managed care

6. *Which of the following is **not** a key element in developing a profile that will allow the physician to prosper financially and make a genuine difference when working with the business community?*

A. gaining a basic foundation in occupational medicine
B. being prepared to address the full occupational medicine continuum
C. associating interventions in terms of health care cost containment
D. resisting the temptation to play multiple roles
E. thinking of oneself as an educator

REFERENCES

McCunney RJ, Barbanel CS. Controlling workers' compensation costs: the role of an audit. *Occup. Health Saf.* 62(10):75, 1993.
Reece R, Coombes D. Clinical corner. *Visions* 3:14, 1993.

9

Drug Testing

OBJECTIVES

- Explain the scope of drug testing in the contemporary workplace
- List the types of work-site drug testing
- Discuss problems involved in specimen collection
- Explain the duties of the Medical Review Officer (MRO)
- Discuss controversial issues concerning drug and alcohol tests

OUTLINE

IX. Current Issues
    A. Individual Privacy Versus Public Health and Safety
    B. Specimen Dilution and Adulteration
    C. MRO Credentialing
    D. Evidence of Drug Testing Effectiveness
    E. Americans with Disabilities Act
    F. On-Site Testing
    G. Choice of Drug Panel
    H. Screening Cutoff Levels
    I. Hair Analysis
 X. Conclusions
XI. References
XII. Appendix to Chapter 9: ACOEM Drug Screening in the Workplace: Ethical Guidelines

KEY POINTS

- The most essential factor responsible for the extraordinary growth of drug testing has been the availability of simple, inexpensive immunoassay urine screening tests. Gas chromatography/mass spectrometry (GC/MS) has become the "gold standard" for forensic drug testing.
- In 1990, companies with more than 250 employees were much more likely to have written policies for drug programs. Drugs in the workplace are a concern because 66.5% of current illicit drug users are employed. Illicit drug use is heavily concentrated among those aged 18 to 34 (9.7% of full-time employees, based on 1991 surveys). Illicit drug use among employees is associated with higher rates of absenteeism, accidental injury, involuntary separation, medical care usage, and health care costs.
- Six major drug testing situations exist: preemployment/preplacement, periodic, postaccident/incident, reasonable cause/reasonable suspicion, return to duty and follow-up, and random. Unannounced random drug testing provides the highest deterrent against drug use.
- There are two categories of drug testing, regulated versus nonregulated.
- Federal regulations contain detailed procedures for urine collection, completion of custody and control forms, analysis by laboratories certified originally by the National Institute on Drug Abuse (NIDA) for only five specified illicit drugs (amphetamines, cocaine, marijuana, opiates, and phencyclidine—the "NIDA-5"), and mandatory reporting of all results to an MRO for review and interpretation before reporting to the employer.
- Most positive drug tests that are invalidated are due to improper urine collection or documentation.
- A minimum of four entries (date, two actual signatures, and courier) must appear in the chain of custody block of the DOT-type form. It is vitally important that the urine collection process treat each person with respect and allow the maximum reasonable privacy, while minimizing the opportunity to substitute or adulterate urine specimens. There are three ways to conduct urine collection: private collection, monitored, and direct observation. Direct observation requires same gender collection site personnel as the donor. The collected sample should remain in constant view of the collector and donor until it has been properly sealed with a tamper-proof seal and labeled. If an employer has requested both a federally mandated drug test and nonregulated testing, separately voided specimens must be collected with separate custody and control forms.
- In the laboratory analysis, if the screen is positive, then another aliquot is taken from the specimen for confirmation testing for the identified drug by gas chromatography/mass spectrometry (GC/MS). Administrative cutoff levels for each of the five

illicit drugs are specified by the regulation for each form of testing (see Table 9–4). When the laboratory identifies a specimen as negative, it is discarded. Positive specimens are frozen and retained at the laboratory for at least one full year in case the analysis is questioned and retests must be performed. Laboratories must retain specimen records for a minimum of 2 years. The DOT has issued guidance to laboratories regarding "fatal flaws" that constitute grounds for rejecting a specimen (see Table 9–3). Some flaws may be corrected by a signed affidavit from the appropriate individual. When repeat analysis is requested or when split samples are tested, only GC/MS confirmation is performed for the analyte that was positive initially at the laboratory's lower limits of detection.

- In unregulated testing, results may go directly to the employer. In federally regulated testing, the results must go to an MRO. Negative laboratory results with a flawed chain of custody section must be reported as a canceled test, rather than negative, unless corrected by signed affidavit. The most critical MRO function is to interpret and verify positive test results. The MRO must allow individuals with positive tests the opportunity to provide a legitimate medical explanation. Guidelines have been developed for the MRO to follow (see Table 9–5).

- MRO verification of legitimate medical explanations for positive tests often requires clinical judgment. For example, although inhalation of sidestream marijuana smoke is offered as an explanation for a positive test result, toxicology studies have not confirmed this explanation as feasible. Ingestion of poppy seeds can cause high levels of urine opiates. Consideration of whether spousal use is legitimate or unauthorized drug use remains an MRO judgment, although DOT recommends that these be verified as positive. Completed custody and control forms should not be used for reporting results to the employer, because many forms will show laboratory positives that, because of legitimate medical use, were verified as negative.

- In the Omnibus Transportation Employee Testing Act of 1991, Congress mandated testing for misuse of alcohol as well as controlled substances in most transportation sectors including intrastate vehicle operators who hold a commercial driver's license (such as school bus drivers). Tests must be conducted using evidential grade breath testing devices approved by the National Highway Transportation Safety Administration (NHTSA). Tests must be conducted by a trained, certified breath alcohol technician (BAT) who has demonstrated proficiency in a NHTSA-approved course. Employees with alcohol concentrations of 0.02 mg% or greater will be removed from safety-sensitive duty, and if the level is 0.04 mg% or greater, return to work will be permitted only after evaluation and rehabilitation.

- Although MRO certification is not required by current federal regulations, the Medical Review Officer Certification Council (MROCC), established in 1992 by ACOEM, offers a rigorous certifying examination following a minimum of 12 hours of approved MRO training.

- Drug testing programs cannot assure a drug-free workplace. The importance of employee assistance programs (EAPs) cannot be overemphasized. Given the dynamic nature of drug testing regulations, the MRO must remain abreast of the most current developments.

- The ACOEM Ethical Guidelines for Drug Screening in the Workplace list several features that should be included in any program for the screening of employees and prospective employees for drugs (see Guidelines).

QUESTIONS

1. *All of the following are usual situations in which drug testing is performed for the work site **except**:*

A. preemployment/preplacement.
B. reassignment to a higher paying position.
C. periodic.

D. postaccident/postincident.
E. random.

2. *Regarding the urine collection process for regulated urine drug testing:*

A. it is vitally important that the urine collection process treat each person with respect and allow the maximum reasonable privacy, while minimizing the opportunity to substitute or adulterate urine specimens.
B. a chain of custody is unimportant.
C. direct observation of the urine exiting the urinary meatus is the only acceptable form of collection.
D. once the sample is handed by the donor to the collector, the donor may leave.
E. a single void may be used to collect samples for both regulated and nonregulated testing.

3. *In reviewing a positive test result with the donor, which of the following is most likely to support a Medical Review Officer (MRO) determination of legitimate use?*

A. Passive inhalation of marijuana smoke at a social gathering
B. Consumption of sesame seeds
C. Use of a spouse's prescription medication
D. A prescription written by a licensed physician
E. Eating deer meat from a buck which consumed wild growth of marijuana

4. *Certification of Medical Review Officers (MROs) is required to participate in authorized drug testing by which of the following organizations:*

A. National Institute for Drug Abuse (NIDA)
B. Medical Review Officer Certification Council
C. Department of Transportation
D. Substance Abuse and Mental Health Services Administration
E. none of the above

5. *The NIDA drugs of abuse covered in the Federal Drug Free Workplace testing program include:*

A. amphetamines, cocaine, opiates, marijuana, and phencyclidine.
B. amphetamines, barbiturates, codeine, marijuana, and phencyclidine.
C. barbiturates, codeine, marijuana, opiates, and pentachlorophenol.
D. barbiturates, cocaine, codeine, methamphetamine, and phencyclidine.
E. amphetamines, barbiturates, benzodiazepines, codeine, and marijuana.

6. *ACOEM Ethical Guidelines for Drug Testing include all of the following **except:***

A. reasonable privacy during specimen collection.
B. advanced employee notification of policy and testing procedures.
C. written informed consent for screening and results notification.
D. notification of donor of positive drug test results.
E. Medical Review Officer review of positive test results.

7. *U.S. Department of Transportation screening cutoffs for alcohol breath testing, for removal from safety-sensitive duty pending evaluation and rehabilitation (if needed), are:*

A.   0.05 mg% screening; 0.04 confirmation.
B.   0.1 mg% screening; 0.05 confirmation.
C.   0.04 mg% screening; 0.02 confirmation.
D.   0.04 mg% on both screening and confirmation.
E.   0.01 mg% on both screening and confirmation.

REFERENCES

Diagnostic Criteria from DSM-III. Washington, DC: American Psychiatric Association, 1982.
Medical Review Officer Certification Council, 55 W. Seegers Rd., Arlington Heights, IL 60005, 708-228-6850.

10

Accreditation of Occupational Health Clinical Centers

OBJECTIVES

- Explain the importance of accreditation of occupational health centers
- List components of the survey process
- Differentiate between the core and adjunct standards required for accreditation

OUTLINE

I. The Accreditation Association for Ambulatory Health Care
II. Accreditation Under AAAHC
III. Survey Eligibility
IV. Survey Process
V. AAAHC Standards
  A. Core Standards
    1. Patient Rights
    2. Governance
    3. Administration
    4. Quality of Care
    5. Quality Assurance
    6. Clinical Records
    7. Professional Improvement
    8. Facilities and Environment
  B. Adjunct Standards
    1. Occupational Health Services
    2. Immediate/Urgent Care Services
    3. Testing: Diagnostic Imaging and Laboratory Services
    4. Other Professional and Technical Services
    5. Other Standards
VI. Problem Areas in Achieving Accreditation
  A. Clinical Records

      B. Quality Assurance
         1. Structure
         2. Content Areas
         3. Quality Assurance Studies
         4. Practice Guidelines
      C. Occupational Health Services
         1. Prevention
         2. Treatment
         3. Regulations
         4. Integration with Other Standards
  VII. Rationale for Accreditation
 VIII. References

KEY POINTS

- Medical organizations may pursue accreditation to improve operations and quality of care as well as for financial reasons, assuring reimbursement through third-party payers, expanding market shares, or reducing insurance premiums. ACOEM supports the development of standards of practice, the achievement of these standards through self-evaluation, and the participation in accreditation to demonstrate that the standards have been met.
- The development of the Accreditation Association for Ambulatory Health Care (AAAHC) as a separate organization was prompted by a reorganization of the Joint Commission for the Accreditation of Hospitals (now the JCAHO). Seeking accreditation is a voluntary process. There are 22 individual standards in AAAHC's handbook, which are divided into two groups: core and adjunct. Core standards apply to all organizations and address issues common to ambulatory health care delivery, such as administration, facilities, and records. Adjunct standards address specific services or activities and only apply if the organization is active in these areas. One of the adjunct standards is occupational health services.
- Eligibility requirements for accreditation surveys include the following:
  - The organization's primary activity must by provision of health services and it must have been in operation for at least 6 months.
  - Either the organization or its parent organization must be a formally organized, legal entity. If required, the organization must be licensed to provide services and be in compliance with appropriate regulations.
  - For occupational health services, medical care must be under the direction or supervision of a physician(s).
  - The health care organization must also share facilities, equipment, and patient care records among its members providing patient care.
- Preparation for an AAAHC survey begins with a self-assessment process including the creation of a committee or team. The process may be lengthy, dependent on the status of the organization. A presurvey questionnaire is completed and submitted. The survey consists of an extensive on-site evaluation of policies, procedures, and operations. A primary goal of the surveyors is to determine if the organization is in compliance with the intent of the standards. A second goal is to educate and provide consultation. Accreditation can be granted for either 1 or 3 years.
- AAAHC has eight core standards: patient rights, governance, administration, quality of care, quality assurance, clinical records, professional improvement, and facilities and environment. A separate adjunct standard exists for occupational health services. The opening statement sets the goals of occupational health services as assuring a safe and healthy workplace through the recognition, evaluation, and control of illness and injury in or from the workplace. The occupational health standard contains several points, focusing on issues such as regulatory compliance, appropriate training, access to reference materials and an occupational health physician, con-

tinuing education, minimizing disability, restoring function, matching medical status with work demand, medical surveillance, and confidentiality. Other applicable adjunct standards may include immediate/urgent care services, testing (both diagnostic imaging and laboratory services), and other professional and technical services (such as occupational therapy, physical therapy, psychological services, health education, and audiology).

- Problems in accreditation are usually in one of three areas: clinical records, quality assurance, or occupational health services.
- Under clinical records, a problem is failing to adequately document the patient encounter. To evaluate care, the medical records must provide sufficient detail so that an outside reviewer can (1) determine the patient's primary complaint, (2) independently confirm the patient's diagnosis based on reported findings, (3) confirm that the treatment was appropriate and necessary, and (4) confirm that the patient's care was appropriate over time. Records must be complete and legible.
- Successful quality assurance programs require commitment and participation from the entire organization, starting with the governing body. All staff must be involved including professional and administrative. Central to the process is the Quality Assurance Study. This study applies research principles to analyze a problem, management principles to implement a corrective change, and surveillance principles to assure that the measure is effective. Practice guidelines are an important element of quality assurance, but some physicians are reluctant to participate in such programs because of concerns over the practice of "cookbook medicine" and application of punitive measures.
- The specific goals of the occupational health services standard should be reflected in all other relevant AAAHC standards. Documentation must include preventive activities, knowledge of the workplace, and compliance with all applicable rules and regulations.

QUESTIONS

*1. All of the following are true regarding accreditation under the AAAHC **except:***

A. accreditation is voluntary.
B. AAAHC is part of the Joint Commission on Accreditation of Healthcare Organizations (JCAHO).
C. there are 22 individual standards, which are divided into two groups: core and adjunct.
D. organizations may be motivated to seek accreditation to improve operations and quality of care.
E. organizations may be motivated to seek accreditation for financial reasons.

*2. Which of the following is **not** an eligibility requirement for AAAHC survey?*

A. For occupational health services, medical care must be under the direction or supervision of a physician(s), certified by the American Board of Preventive Medicine in Occupational Medicine.
B. The organization's primary activity must be provision of health services.
C. The organization must have been in operation for at least 6 months.
D. The organization or its parent organization must be a formally organized, legal entity.
E. The health care organization must share facilities, equipment, and patient care records among its members providing patient care.

3. The AAAHC survey process:

A. usually requires the dedication of a single employee.

B. is normally conducted by telephone and modem.
C. is intended primarily to assess compliance with OSHA regulations.
D. offers as a goal education of and consultation to the surveyed organization.
E. results in accreditation for 5 years.

4. *All of the following topics represent AAAHC core standards* **except:**

A. patient rights.
B. quality assurance.
C. clinical records.
D. professional improvement.
E. billing.

5. *The occupational health services adjunct standard of AAAHC provides for all of the following* **except:**

A. health care providers must have access to reference materials and an occupational health physician.
B. confidential information may be provided to employers as long as they are representatives of human resources.
C. medical management includes consideration of the relationship of the patient's condition to work.
D. medical care should strive to minimize disability and restore function as soon as possible.
E. preplacement examinations must consider both the patient's medical status and the work demands.

6. *In order for AAAHC to evaluate patient care, medical records must provide sufficient detail so that an outside reviewer can perform all of the following* **except:**

A. estimate the complexity of the visit to establish the level of service rendered.
B. determine the patient's primary complaint.
C. independently confirm the patient's diagnosis based on reported findings.
D. confirm that the treatment was appropriate and necessary.
E. confirm that the patient's care was appropriate over time.

7. *Practice guidelines:*

A. are intended to serve as menus for conducting patient care.
B. are developed as punitive tools to control utilization of resources by physicians.
C. are protocols intended solely for training medical students.
D. attempt to create a template for the best quality care for patients.
E. should be changed only once every 3 to 5 years.

Section 1 Answers

CHAPTER 1 ANSWERS

1. The answer is B. (Reference: pp. 3–4)

The history of occupational medicine can be traced back to antiquity. Observations related to increased rates of illnesses and mortality among miners date back to Roman times; however, explanations for this phenomenon were often attributed to the fact that workers were slaves and thus of a more feeble constitution. It was not until the late seventeenth century, when an Italian physician published *Disease and Occupations,* that physicians were formally urged to pay attention to the role of one's work in the development of certain illnesses.

Although occupational medicine has been a distinct discipline within the American Board of Preventive Medicine since 1954, a considerable shortage of well-trained and certified specialists in this field exists. In large part, this shortage is due to a deficiency of postgraduate training positions. The situation is now changing.

A relatively unknown fact is that over 90% of businesses in the United States and the world have over 100 or fewer employees. It is rarely economically feasible for these enterprises to provide anything other than meager health care and, in some cases, at best first aid.

2. The answer is E. (Reference: p. 9)

Ancillary services refer to laboratory and related procedures conducted as part of clinical evaluations. The type and level of ancillary services depend on the practice setting and the local medical community. In the provision of occupational health services to small businesses, however, the following items are considered essential: an audiometric booth and audiometer, a well-functioning and calibrated spirometer, and a vision screener. Optional services include laboratory, x-ray, and physical therapy; however, the appropriateness of including these services will vary. In some cases, it may be suitable to employ referral services.

3. The answer is C. (Reference: pp. 14, 15)

The goals of an occupational health service include the following:
A. To protect people at work from health and safety hazards
B. To protect the local environment
C. To facilitate safe placement of workers according to their physical, mental, and emotional capacities
D. To assure adequate medical care and rehabilitation of the occupationally ill and injured
E. To assist in measures related to personal maintenance

4. The answer is E. (Reference: Tables 1–1, 1–2; p. 5)

5. The answer is A. (Reference: p. 6)

The physician conducting a preplacement evaluation has an obligation to the business enterprise to report functional limitations and corresponding accommodations that may be necessary to work. The physician should pay heed to medical confidentiality on non–work-related illnesses. Although the criteria used to define health conditions that fall under this category may be blurred at times, the physician should strive to be recognized as impartial in these often difficult settings. Ideally, the patient should be advised as to what information will be released to the employer. Similarly, as part of this process, it is advisable that a person undergoing a preplacement evaluation sign an appropriate release form that allows the physician to discuss pertinent medical findings with the business.

Medical records should not be released to the business unless an on-site medical office is maintained and supervised by a registered nurse or physician who can assume responsibility for the ethical maintenance of the medical records.

Table 1-1. *Occupational and environmental health programs: essential components*

1. Health evaluation of employees
    A. Preassignment
    B. Medical surveillance
    C. Post illness or injury
2. Diagnosis and treatment of occupational and environmental injuries or illnesses, including rehabilitation
3. Emergency treatment of nonoccupational injury or illness
4. Education of employees and jobs where potential occupational hazards exist
5. Implementation of programs for personal protective equipment
6. Evaluation, inspection, and abatement of workplace hazards
7. Toxicologic assessments, including advice on chemical substances that have not had adequate toxicologic testing
8. Biostatistics and epidemiology assessments
9. Maintenance of occupational medical records
10. Immunization against possible occupational infections
11. Medical interpretation and participation in governmental health and safety regulations
12. Periodic evaluation of the occupational or environmental health program
13. Disaster preparedness: planning for the workplace and community
14. Assistance in rehabilitation of alcohol- and drug-dependent employees or those with emotional disorders

Source: Adapted from Scope of occupational and environmental health programs and practices, report of the Occupational Medical Practice Committee of the American College of Occupational and Environmental Medicine. *J. Occup. Med.* 34:436, 1992.

Table 1-2. *Elective components of occupational and environmental health programs*

1. Palliative treatment of nonoccupational disorders
2. Repetitive treatment of nonoccupational conditions prescribed and monitored by personal physicians
3. Assistance and control of illness-related job absenteeism
4. Assistance and evaluation of personal health care
5. Immunizations against nonoccupational infectious diseases
6. Health education and counseling
7. Termination and retirement administration
8. Participation in planning and assessing of the quality of employee health benefits
9. Participation and systematic research

Source: Adapted from Scope of occupational and environmental health programs and practices, report of the Occupational Medical Practice Committee of the American College of Occupational and Environmental Medicine. *J. Occup. Med.* 34:436, 1992.

CHAPTER 2 ANSWERS

1. The answer is C. (Reference: pp. 20, 21)

Until the early years of the twentieth century, if employees were injured in their place of employment, the only remedy against the employer was a suit at common law.

In the early twentieth century, employers and employees in the various states began to make a deal. That deal was known as workers' compensation. The workers' compensation statutes varied a bit from state to state (each state has its own workers' compensation law), but each is composed of several compromises:

1. Employees gave up their right to sue employers at common law and agreed to accept a certain sum of money per week for their inability to work as a result of work-related injuries. They agreed to accept this compensation as their exclusive remedy against the employer.
2. Employers agreed to give injured employees a certain sum of money per week, if they were unable to work as a result of work-related injuries. Thus, payment would be made, regardless of fault.
3. Payment would be automatic unless disputes arose. The disputes over issues of work-relatedness, amounts of entitlement, timeliness of claim, etc., would (generally) be decided by administrative bodies, rather than courts.
4. Payments would only be made for disability (i.e., inability to work).[1] No damages would be allowed as a punishment of the employer (punitive damages).

At first, most of the state workers' compensation systems covered only work-related accidents. Illness and disease coverage were added later.

2. The answer is B. (Reference: p. 23)

In recent years, many states and OSHA have enacted rules mandating that employees be provided with information about the chemical exposures they are receiving in the workplace and how those exposures may affect their health. OSHA's rule is known as the Hazard Communication Standard (HCS) [29 CFR]. The HCS originally covered only entities in the manufacturing sector and importers of chemicals.

Because of the potential for conflicting regulations, OSHA expanded the coverage of the HCS to all employers covered by the OSH Act.

Generally, the HCS requires that:

1. Containers in the workplace that contain hazardous chemicals[2] must be labeled with the chemical's identity, appropriate hazard warnings, and the identity of the manufacturer.
2. Employees must be trained about the hazards of chemicals to which they are or may be exposed.
3. Material Safety Data Sheets (MSDS), which set out in considerable detail the hazards of specific chemicals, must be made available to employees who may be exposed to those chemicals.

3. The answer is A. (Reference: p. 24, Table 2–1)

---

1. Most state laws did contain scheduled awards, in which a certain percentage of impairment resulted in a certain payment of compensation, even though the employee continued to work. Thus, loss of a finger or partial loss of vision or hearing might result in payment of a number of weeks of compensation, even though it did not affect ability to work.

2. Hazardous chemicals are defined in the HCS as being those chemicals that present one of several physical hazards (e.g., flammability, reactivity, or explosiveness) or a health hazard. Health hazards include carcinogens, mutagens, teratogens, and toxins to any of the body's organ systems [29 CFR 1910.1200(c), (d)]. A determination as to what constitutes a hazard must be made by the manufacturer or importer, but downstream users may also make that determination [29 CFR 1910.1200(d)(1), (2)].

Table 2–1. *Information provided on material safety Data Sheets (MSDS)*

1. The label identity of the chemical
2. The chemical and common names including synonyms
3. If the substance is a mixture that has been tested as a whole to determine its hazards, the chemical and common names of the ingredients that contribute to the known hazards
4. If the substance is a mixture that has not been tested as a whole, the chemical and common names of all ingredients that have been determined to be health hazards and that constitute 1% or more of the mixture (or 0.1% or more, if the hazard is a carcinogen)
5. The chemical and common names of all ingredients that have been determined to present a physical hazard
6. The physical and chemical characteristics of the chemical
7. The physical hazards of the chemical
8. The health hazards of the chemical, including signs and symptoms of exposure, and any medical conditions that can be aggravated by exposure to the chemical
9. The primary routes of exposure
10. The OSHA permissible exposure limit, the American Conference of Governmental Industrial Hygienists (ACGIH) threshold limit value, or any other recommended exposure limit
11. Whether the substance is listed on the National Toxicology Program's "Annual List of Carcinogens" or has been found to be a potential carcinogen by the International Agency for Research on Cancer or OSHA
12. Known precautions for safe handling and use
13. Applicable control measures
14. The date of preparation of the latest MSDS or its latest change
15. The name, address, and telephone number of the manufacturer, importer, employer, or other responsible party preparing or distributing the MSDS, who can provide additional information on the hazardous chemical and appropriate emergency procedures

4. The answer is C. (Reference: p. 27)

The OSHA 200 Log is used to record the occurrence and extent of occupational injuries and illnesses, and at the end of the year it is used to summarize the injuries and illnesses that occurred during the year. Each injury or illness must be classified as either (1) a death case, (2) a case involving lost workdays (which includes days of restricted work activity as well as days off work), or (3) a case not involving lost workdays. In addition, for occupational illnesses, the log must record whether the illness was a skin disorder, a dust disease of the lungs, a respiratory condition caused by a toxic agent, systemic poisoning, a disorder due to repeated trauma or physical agents, or another type of occupational illness. New entries should not be made on the OSHA 200 Log if the employee is merely experiencing a recurrence of symptoms from an earlier injury or illness.

The OSHA Form 200 must be maintained for 5 calendar years following the year to which it relates.

Employee access to the OSHA 200 Log is limited to the logs for the establishment where the employee worked or formerly worked.

All employers must report to OSHA, within 48 hours, accidents that result in one or more deaths or in the hospitalization of five or more employees.

5. The answer is D. (Reference: pp. 28, 29)

By its terms, OSHA's Record Access Standard "applies to all employee exposure and medical records, and analyses thereof, made or maintained in any manner, including on an in-house or contractual (fee-for-service) basis."

Under the Record Access Standard, any employer who has employees exposed to "toxic substances" or "harmful physical agents" must provide the employee (or his or her authorized representative) access to his or her medical record within 15 days of a request.

This provision applies to all present and former employees exposed to toxic substances or harmful physical agents. All medical records must be retained for the duration of the employee's employment plus 30 years.

To obtain access to medical records, any designated representatives must have the written consent of the employee.

Any authorizations expire after 1 year.

There is one circumstance under which a physician for the employer may prohibit an employee from seeing his or her medical record. If the physician believes that direct employee access to records concerning a terminal illness or a psychiatric condition of that employee could be detrimental to the employee's health, the employer may refuse to show these records to the employee. However, the records must be shown to the employee's authorized representative.

6. The answer is C. (Reference: pp. 30–34)

With regard to preplacement or periodic examinations, physicians should be aware of the code of Ethical Conduct of the American College of Occupational and Environmental Medicine, originally adopted in 1976 and updated in 1994: "Employers are entitled to counsel about the medical fitness of individuals in relation to work, but are not entitled to diagnoses or details of a specific nature."

Under the ADA a disability is (1) a physical or mental impairment that substantially limits one or more of the major life activities of an individual, (2) a record of such an impairment, or (3) a situation in which an individual is regarded as having such an impairment. The thrust of the ADA (relevant to employers) is that employees or job applicants with such disabilities may not be discriminated against in any aspect of the employment relationship if that employee or applicant is qualified for the job. A disabled person is qualified if, with reasonable accommodation, he or she can perform the essential functions of the job as well as one who is not disabled.

The toxic tort is another possible concern for the practitioner of occupational medicine. Toxic tort suits are suits at common law, brought by those who claim that exposure to the toxic substance caused them some injury or disorder. Normally, but not always (see the exception to workers' compensation exclusivity for intentional torts), workers' compensation will be the sole remedy for employees harmed by exposure to toxic substances at the workplace that are being manufactured by their own employer. However, workers can always sue third-party suppliers of materials (e.g., asbestos) to their employers. Consumers of products (e.g., pharmaceuticals such as diethylstilbestrol) or those exposed to allegedly toxic waste in the environment (e.g., a Superfund site) can also bring a civil suit.

Practitioners of occupational medicine need no longer concern themselves with monitoring or enforcing fetal protection programs, since the Supreme Court recently found such programs to be unlawfully discriminatory. Fetal protection programs directed solely at women and solely for the protection of fetuses are not legitimate employer policies.

Most challenges to private employer drug testing have been based on common-law privacy interests. Most of these cases have involved testing of employees in safety-sensitive jobs and, predictably, testing has been upheld. As in the federal Fourth Amendment cases, the courts usually have reached their conclusions by balancing employee privacy expectations against employer interest in safety.

The propriety of testing is most uncertain where employers wish to test employees in nonsensitive positions.

CHAPTER 3 ANSWERS

1. The answer is B. (Reference: pp. 38–41)

The OSH Act does not cover federal, state, or local municipal employees. However, executive branches of the federal government are expected to have equivalent regulations and most state-run programs cover state and local municipal employees.

This OSHA standard requires annual examinations for employees exposed to noise of 85 dBA or higher on a daily time-weighted average (TWA) basis.

In general, the OSHA standards require the physician to furnish the employer a written opinion on whether the employee has any medical conditions that would place the employee at increased risk of impairment from the work or use of protective equipment. The physician must provide in writing any limitations on the employee's assigned work. The employee should be informed of any conditions that require further examination or treatment and be referred to private physicians, as necessary.

There are detailed individual standards for 26 chemicals. Each of these standards includes a section on medical surveillance. In all standards, medical examinations are required if certain conditions are met.

Some of the more recent standards also include provisions for medical removal protection and multiple physician review (e.g., lead [1910.1025] and methylene dianiline [1910.1050]). In some cases, the criteria for medical removal may be straightforward. In lead exposure, for example, temporary removal from exposure is required if the average of the last three blood tests for lead is greater than 50 g/100 g whole blood and the last test is over 40 g/100 g whole blood.

2. The answer is D. (Reference: p. 39, 40)

An injury that requires only first-aid care as opposed to medical treatment is not recordable. In contrast, all illnesses are recordable regardless of how trivial they may be. Employers greatly appreciate injuries being given first aid rather than medical treatment whenever this level of care is sufficient. OSHA also has definitions of what is first aid and what is medical treatment. For example, use of over-the-counter medication is first aid, use of prescription medication is medical treatment. Likewise, use of a Band-Aid is first aid, whereas use of a Steri-Strip is considered medical treatment. For minor injuries, the selection of treatment can determine OSHA recordability.

Records must be maintained for the duration of a person's employment plus 30 years. This time period is much longer than that typically required for non–work-related inactive patient files. OSHA also requires that medical records be released to designated representatives, including the employee, on presentation of signed consent. Compliance with such requests is required within 15 working days (Doyle, 1989).

Audiograms that show a standard threshold shift (STS), which is defined as an age-adjusted decrease of 10 dB or greater in either ear averaged for the frequencies of 2,000, 3,000, and 4,000 Hz, must be evaluated by an audiologist or physician to determine the need for further evaluation.

Based on current OSHA field directives, a work-related change in hearing of 25 dB averaged over the frequencies of 2,000, 3,000, and 4,000 Hz must be recorded on the OSHA Form 200 as a disorder due to repeated trauma.

3. The answer is B. (Reference: Table 3–3, p. 39)

4. The answer is A. (Reference: pp. 38, 40, 41)

Some states have taken advantage of an option in the OSH Act to establish and administer their own state OSHA plan. Standards promulgated by these states are usually identical to the federal OSHA standards but in some cases may be more stringent.

Table 3–3. *OSHA chemical specific standards*

Section no.[a]	Chemical
1910.1001	Asbestos
1910.1003	4-Nitrobiphenyl
1910.1004	Alpha-Naphthylamine
1910.1006	Methyl chlormethyl ether
1910.1007	3,3'-Dichlorobenzidine (and its salts)
1910.1008	bis-Chloromethyl ether
1910.1009	beta-Naphylamine
1910.1010	Benzidine
1910.1011	4-Aminodiphenyl
1910.1012	Ethylenimine
1910.1013	beta-Propiolactone
1910.1014	2-Acetylaminofluorene
1910.1015	2-Dimethylaminoazobenzene
1910.1016	N-Nitrosodimethylamine
1910.1017	Vinyl chloride
1910.1018	Inorganic arsenic
1910.1025	Lead
1910.1027	Cadmium
1910.1028	Benzene
1910.1029	Coke-oven emissions
1910.1043	Cotton dust
1910.1044	1,2 dibromo 3-chloropropane
1910.1045	Acrylonitrile
1910.1047	Ethylene oxide
1910.1048	Formaldehyde
1910.1050	Methylene dianiline

[a]From title 29 of the code of Federal Regulations.

Injuries and illnesses are recorded on an OSHA Form 200 by the employer. The threshold of recordability is different depending on whether the case is an injury or illness. These terms are defined differently by OSHA than they have been traditionally defined in medicine. OSHA's definition of an injury is something that is caused by an instantaneous exposure, for example in the snap of the fingers. An illness is anything caused by a longer exposure even if it is as short as a couple of seconds.

Several OSHA standards, including Hazardous Waste Operations and Emergency Response, Respiratory Protection, and some Chemical Specific Standards, require the employee to have a medical examination to determine physical fitness to perform certain jobs, or to wear specific personal protective equipment (e.g., respirators).

None of these standards specifies details of the medical examination, which are left to the discretion of the examining physician. Employers may specify requirements.

OSHA's standard on blood-borne pathogens is directly primarily at the health care industry, but also affects blood processing and research activities using human blood or other bodily fluids, as well as any employer that has designated first-aid responders.

5. The answer is D. (Reference: p. 42)

The National Institute for Occupational Safety and Health is the research agency created by the OSH Act. In 1973, NIOSH became part of the CDC. The institute is mandated to protect the health and safety of workers by conducting research on workplace hazards.

NIOSH plays an important role in providing information pertinent to the development of OSHA standards. Before making specific recommendations, NIOSH performs research and conducts a literature review of human and animal literature and other test systems.

At either employee or employer request, NIOSH may conduct a Health Hazard Evaluation (HHE), which includes an industrial hygiene study and appropriate medical evaluation of an occupational health problem.

The majority of the training and educational services provided by NIOSH are conducted at 15 Education Resource Centers (ERCs), which were established in 1977 because of the shortage of occupational health professionals. A variety of programs are offered, including occupational medicine residencies and graduate school training in occupational nursing, industrial hygiene, and safety.

6. The answer is C. (Reference: pp. 43–45)

NIOSH develops health standards for MSHA, but only advises OSHA concerning health standards.

Regulations issued by the NRC require that a physician determine a worker's ability to wear a respirator every 12 months. This is in contrast to OSHA's standard, in which an annual review is suggested but longer time intervals are acceptable.

The Equal Employment Opportunity Commission (EEOC) is charged with enforcing the Americans with Disabilities Act.

The Toxic Substance Control Act (TSCA): Section 8c of this act requires manufacturers or users of a specific chemical to keep a record of any allegation of a heretofore unknown adverse health effect.

TSCA requires manufacturers, producers, and users of chemicals to report to the EPA new information that reasonably supports the conclusion that the chemical or mixture presents a substantial risk of injury to health or the environment.

ATSDR is primarily concerned with the potential adverse health effects associated with environmental exposure to toxic substances. ATSDR's mission is to support activities designed to protect the public from the adverse health consequences of toxic chemical exposure.

Part of its mission is to conduct research about the health effects of toxic materials.

ATSDR is mandated to establish a disease and exposure registry to provide an information base of health effects of toxic substances. It also provides continuing education training for physicians through case studies in environmental medicine.

CHAPTER 4 ANSWERS

1. The answer is B. (Reference: Table 4–1, p. 49)

2. The answer is B. (Reference: pp. 50, 53)

Prevention has particular value in the design and operation of programs since all occupational medical problems are potentially preventable. Public health professionals use the principles of prevention in their daily development of programs. Prevention has three components: primary, secondary, and tertiary. Primary prevention is any intervention that addresses a risk factor for a disease or injury. Examples include immunization against infectious diseases and reduction in blood cholesterol levels to reduce the risk of heart disease and stroke. Secondary prevention refers to early detection of disease and intervention before symptoms appear. The goal is to reverse, halt, or retard the progression of a disorder. Examples include the use of mammography in the early detection of breast cancer and periodic cytologic testing of the uterine cervix (Papanicolaou smear) in screening for cervical cancer. Tertiary prevention refers to minimizing the effects of disease and disability by reducing complications and premature deterioration. Examples include the care of pressure points and bladder function in bedridden individuals. Traditionally, occupational health programs (both company based and contract services) limited their role to tertiary prevention—the management of occupational injury and illness. Recently, there has been a much greater emphasis on programs addressing primary and secondary prevention. With the increasing costs of workers compensation, these programs should have a greater emphasis.

3. The answer is A. (Reference: p. 53)

Biologic monitoring is an attempt to assess the internal dose of overall worker exposure to chemicals in the workplace through measurement of the appropriate determinant in biologic specimens such as urine, blood, or exhaled air. The American Conference of Governmental Industrial Hygienists (ACGIH) has developed biologic exposure indices (BEIs) that are intended as guidelines for analyzing the results of biologic monitoring (American College of Industrial Hygienists, 1991). High body fluid levels that suggest overexposure to chemicals should prompt a work-site evaluation by an industrial hygienist. Low levels tend to indicate a healthy working environment, help to establish confidence among workers, and reduce frivolous lawsuits. Although biologic monitoring may or may not be part of a medical surveillance program, it has advantages over air monitoring, including the following:

It takes into account absorption via routes other than inhalation.

Table 4–1. *Guidelines for the physician conducting a facility walk-through*

1. Are there substances used in the workplace for which established OSHA standards exist?
2. Are carcinogenic substances used?
3. Are corporate policies in effect for certain issues such as alcohol or drug abuse?
4. Are rehabilitative or modified duty assignments available?
5. Are collective bargaining agreements in place that may affect delivery of medical care?
6. Are Material Safety Data Sheets available?
7. What is the level of existing first-aid services?
8. Is a disaster plan in place?
9. What is the nature of control measures (e.g., engineering devices, personal protective equipment)?
10. What staff members are responsible for health and safety measures?
11. What training procedures are in place (regarding Hazard Communication Standard, respiratory use, etc.)?
12. Review current facilities, especially storage of medical records

The substances measured in body fluids relate more directly to an adverse health effect than any environmental measurement.
Personal hygiene habits (such as hand washing, smoking, etc.) are considered.
Individual variation in physiologic parameters, such as respiratory rate (which may alter the amount of exposure measured by air monitoring), are addressed.
Environmental monitoring is not always feasible.

4. The answer is E. (Reference: pp. 55, 56)

Maintaining an on-site program can be a cost-effective method of delivering occupational health services for many organizations, depending on the number of employees and the complexity and health risks of the operations.

In many industries, an occupational health nurse, nurse practitioner, and/or physician assistance provide cost-effective occupational health services. At times, these professionals are also responsible for the assessment and management of workplace health and safety programs and coordinating the off-site services. Responsibilities include tracking injured or ill employees, maintaining the OSHA 200 Log, and delivering a variety of other health- and safety-related prevention programs. If appropriately trained, the professional may also provide supervised clinical care for both work-related and non–work-related medical problems, such as performing preplacement medical surveillance examinations. State regulations vary, however, regarding the degree of autonomy and level of physician supervision that are necessary. In some cases, nurse practitioners and physician assistants may function independently and prescribe medications.

A physician, preferably with certification or training in occupational medicine, is usually necessary. The physician provides medical direction to the staff on the management of work injury and illness, medical surveillance, preplacement, and fitness-for-duty examinations. The physician should be an active member of the team, keep the staff up to date on new regulations, and perform medical review officer–related activities, where appropriate.

The delivery of occupational health care at the workplace can be enhanced by the availability of the rehabilitation staff, including physical therapists and occupational (hand) therapists.

When a business chooses to provide the majority of occupational and medical services on site, adequate space is essential. Ideally, the facility should be in a central area, easily accessed by employees, and kept clean and quiet, especially the hearing booth. Privacy should also be ensured. Good lighting and ventilation are necessary as well as wide doors to allow passage of stretchers and wheelchairs.

5. The answer is E. (Reference: p. 57)

The three primary routes of exposure to hazardous materials are inhalation, ingestion, and skin contact.

Materials can be ingested in the form of aerosols, liquids, or solids. Eating, drinking, or smoking in the work area increases the likelihood of ingestion, as does poor personal hygiene.

Materials can contact the skin in any form. Such materials may be inert, cause local irritation but fail to penetrate the skin, penetrate the skin without local effects, or both irritate and penetrate the skin. Some materials can be absorbed through the skin directly into the bloodstream.

6. The answer is C. (Reference: p. 57)

Materials can be inhaled if they are present in the form of a gas, a vapor, or an aerosol. The word *aerosol* refers to dusts (formed from suspending finely divided solids in air), mists (droplet clouds), fumes (formed from the condensation or reaction products of a gas), and combinations of these types, such as smokes. Gases and vapors may be absorbed from the deep lung directly into the bloodstream, may irritate or damage the respiratory tract at any point, or may condense or react with the moisture in the breath to form an aerosol. Aerosols entering the respiratory tract, or produced there, deposit at locations primarily determined by size (Hatch and Gross, 1964). The largest tend to deposit in the nose and pharynx. Medium-sized aerosols, below 10 μm in diameter, tend to deposit in the nose, pharynx, trachea, and bronchi. Fine aerosols, below about 5 μm in diameter, deposit throughout the respiratory tract, including the deep lung.

CHAPTER 5 ANSWERS

1. The answer is B. (Reference: p. 62, Table 5–1)

2. The answer is E. (Reference: Table 5–1)

The ADA provides limited protection to alcoholics and former drug users who have the disability of addiction. The critical distinction for illegal drug users is between current and former use. Current drug use is defined as use recently enough to justify an employer's reasonable belief that involvement with drugs is an ongoing problem. The

---

Table 5–1. *Definitions from the Americans with Disabilities Act*

Disability (with respect to an individual)
1. A physical or mental impairment that substantially limits one or more of the major life activities of such individual,
2. A record of such an impairment, or
3. Being regarded as having an impairment

Physical or mental impairment
1. Any physiologic disorder or condition, cosmetic disfigurement, or anatomic loss that affects one or more of the following body systems: neurologic, musculoskeletal, special sense organs, respiratory (including speech organs), cardiovascular, reproductive, digestive, genitourinary, hemic and lymphatic, skin and endocrine; or
2. Any mental or psychological disorder, such as mental retardation, organic brain syndrome, emotional or mental illness, and specific learning disabilities

Major life activities
Functions such as caring for oneself, performing manual tasks, walking, seeing, hearing, speaking, breathing, learning, and working

Substantial limits
1. Unable to perform a major life activity that the average person in the general population can perform, or
2. Significantly restricted as to the condition, manner, or duration under which an individual can perform a particular major life activity as compared to the ... average person in the general population

Qualified individual with a disability
An individual with a disability who satisfies the requisite skill, experience, education, and other job-related requirements of the employment position such individual holds or desires, and who, with or without reasonable accommodation, can perform the essential functions of such position

Reasonable accommodation
Modifications or adjustments
1. To a job application process that enable a qualified applicant with a disability to be considered for the position; or
2. To the work environment, or to the manner or circumstances under which the position held or desired is customarily performed, that enable a qualified individual with a disability to perform the essential functions of that position; or
3. That enable a covered entity's employee with a disability to enjoy equal benefits and privileges of employment as are enjoyed by its other similarly situated employees without disabilities

Direct threat
A significant risk of substantial harm to the health or safety of the individual or others that cannot be eliminated or reduced by reasonable accommodation. The determination that an individual poses a "direct threat" shall be based on an individualized assessment of the individual's present ability to safely perform the essential functions of the job. The assessment shall be based on a reasonable medical judgment that relies on the most current medical knowledge and/or on the best available objective evidence. In determining whether an individual would pose a direct threat, the factors to be considered include:
1. The duration of the risk,
2. The nature and severity of the potential harm,
3. The likelihood that the potential harm will occur, and
4. The imminence of the potential harm

Source: From Equal employment opportunities for individuals with disabilities. EEOC; Final Rule. Federal Register 56(144):35735, July 26, 1991.

time is not limited by days or weeks, but must be determined on a case-by-case basis. Former users of illegal drugs are protected if they have completed a supervised rehabilitation program, which can include self-help programs such as Narcotics Anonymous; are participating in a drug rehabilitation program and are not currently using drugs illegally; or were erroneously regarded as using illegal drugs.

3. The answer is E. (Reference: Table 5–1) (See above)

4. The answer is A. (Reference: Table 5–1) (See above)

5. The answer is E. (Reference: pp. 68, 70, 71)

Examinations of employees are limited in scope/content because they must be job-related and consistent with business necessity, or required by federal law. Fitness-for-duty examinations/inquiries must be tailored to measure an employee's ability to perform the essential functions of his/her job. Therefore, it would be inappropriate for an employer to require broad medical histories in cases where such histories are not job-related and consistent with business necessity or are not federally required. In addition, medical histories taken pursuant to a federally required examination must be required for the examination. In short, an employer may not ask disability-related questions as part of a medical history that are broader than required for the examination.

Testing for illegal drugs is specifically excluded as being a medical test. The schedule of drugs is broader than those covered by the Department of Health and Human Services (DHHS) drug testing regulations, and includes any drug that is unlawful under the five schedules of the Controlled Substance Act. Therefore, tests for illicit drugs may be conducted before a job offer. However, an interesting gray area still exists. The EEOC had not considered that, in the case of a positive laboratory test, medical review officers (see Chapter 9) must inquire about legitimate explanations. The Department of Transportation (DOT) considers the medical review officer's function to be an integral part of drug testing, thus excluded from coverage under the ADA. The EEOC has recommended informally that employers arrange drug testing so that any associated medical inquiry is conducted after a conditional job offer has been made. It is also not clear whether alcohol testing, which will be required by DOT regulations, will also be excluded as a medical test (see Chapter 9).

The ADA provides limited protection to alcoholics and former drug users who have the disability of addiction. The critical distinction for illegal drug users is between current and former use. Current drug use is defined as use recently enough to justify an employer's reasonable belief that involvement with drugs is an ongoing problem. The time is not limited by days or weeks, but must be determined on a case-by-case basis. Former users of illegal drugs are protected if they have completed a supervised rehabilitation program, which can include self-help programs such as Narcotics Anonymous; are participating in a drug rehabilitation program and are not currently using drugs illegally; or were erroneously regarded as using illegal drugs.

Alcoholics, while having a disability and being entitled to a reasonable accommodation, may be disciplined or discharged where alcohol use adversely affects job performance or conduct to the extent that the person is no longer qualified for the job. However, the same performance standard must be applied to other employees in the same position. Employers are not required to provide alcohol/drug rehabilitation as a reasonable accommodation.

6. The answer is C. (Reference: p. 64)

Fitness for duty must be individually determined, taking into consideration the nature of the individual's disability and the nature of the individual's job. Medical fitness and risk evaluation can best be achieved by the examiner having intimate familiarity with the essential job functions, frequency and importance of job tasks/demands, and workplace environment (e.g., exposures, use of personal protective equipment, emergency procedures).

7. The answer is D. (Reference: pp. 60, 68)

The ADA prohibits medical examinations in the preemployment phase, allowing them only after a bona fide job offer has been made, and even then only when all employees within a job category are required to have a medical examination.

Because all employees within a job category must be treated the same, if one has a medical inquiry, all must have some kind of medical inquiry. If one has a medical examination, all must have some kind of medical examination. However, the inquiries or examinations do not have to be identical. Therefore, screening questions can be used, for example, "Do you or have you ever had any problems with back pain that restricted your activity?" An examiner may go into detail for those who answer affirmatively. Similarly, positive screening tests may be followed by more definitive ones on a case-by-case basis.

8. The answer is C. (Reference: pp. 68, 69)

The ADA is one of the first federal laws to strongly reinforce confidentiality of medical records. Specifically, it calls for information obtained from medical inquiries or medical examinations to be collected and maintained on separate forms, and to be kept in separate medical files. Confidential medical records are to be maintained by the employer in locked cabinets, separate from personnel files, accessible only to designated persons. Access to this confidential medical information is limited to five situations: (1) informing supervisors and managers about necessary work restrictions and accommodations; (2) informing first-aid and safety personnel, as necessary, if a disability might require emergency treatment (e.g., limited mobility, epilepsy, or diabetes); (3) providing government officials investigating compliance with relevant information on request; (4) providing relevant information to state workers compensation offices or second-injury funds; and (5) providing relevant information to insurance companies that require a medical examination to provide employee health or life insurance.

The applicant/employee should sign a medical release authorizing the dissemination of certain medical information. The ADA requires health professionals to share sufficient information for employers to make management decisions about the presence of a disability, a direct threat to health or safety, and reasonable accommodation.

CHAPTER 6 ANSWERS

1. The answer is B. (Reference: p. 83)

The Code of Ethics of the American Association of Occupational Health Nurses provides guidance for ethical decision making and addresses the following areas:

Provision of nondiscriminatory health care in the work environment with regard for human dignity
Collaboration with other health professionals/agencies to meet the needs of the work force
Protection of the employee's right to privacy and protection of confidential information
Provision of quality care and monitoring of unethical/illegal actions
Acceptance of accountability for health care actions
Maintenance of individual competence
Participation in knowledge-building activities such as research

2. The answer is B. (Reference: p. 81)

The practice of occupational health nursing is defined by the American Association of Occupational Health Nurses as the application of nursing principles in conserving the health of workers in all occupations. It emphasizes prevention, recognition, and treatment of illnesses and injuries, and requires special skills and knowledge in the fields of health education and counseling, environmental health, rehabilitation, and human relations (AAOHN, 1987). The ultimate goal of the nurse in the occupational health setting is to improve, maintain, and restore the health of the worker.

3. The answer is A. (Reference: pp. 79–80)

The occupational health nurse clinician/practitioner applies the nursing process (i.e., assessment, diagnosis, planning, implementation, and evaluation) in providing nursing care for occupational and nonoccupational health problems. Depending on individual knowledge, training, and experience, as well as the legal scope of the licensing authority, the occupational health nurse clinician/practitioner may perform the following major activities:

Assess the work environment for actual and/or potential health hazards
Collect data about the health status of the worker, through an occupational health history, physical assessment, and appropriate laboratory measurements
Develop a nursing diagnosis to formulate a plan of nursing care in collaboration with the employee and other health care professionals, as appropriate
Record health data and maintain accurate employee health records
Provide counseling for worker health problems, health promotion, and disease prevention interventions (e.g., immunization, respiratory protection, hypertension screening, hearing conservation programs)
Develop liaison relationships with community health care providers and organizations for worker health enhancement (e.g., referral to private providers and nonprofit and governmental agencies)

4. The answer is C. (Reference: p. 83)

The occupational health nurse should collaborate with community groups and organizations to develop a network of resources. For example, agencies such as the American Heart Association, American Lung Association, or American Cancer Association can offer valuable materials, information, and expertise to help with health programs or referrals, or both. In addition, working with health departments and hospitals in relation to employee return to work can be mutually beneficial to the company and worker.

5. The answer is C. (Reference: p. 80)

The occupational health nurse administrator provides direction for the planning, implementation, and evaluation of occupational health nursing services. To accomplish this task, the administrator must collaborate with others and facilitate interpersonal relationships for the smooth running of the organizational unit. The occupational health nurse administrator performs the following major activities:

Assesses the health needs of the work force to help plan and develop cost-effective health services

Defines goals and objectives for the occupational health nursing service

Determines resources, such as facilities, staff, and operating expenses, necessary to accomplish unit goals; develops an appropriate, realistic budget; and develops policies and procedures aimed at fostering goal attainment and work performance

Provides nursing leadership in the management and evaluation of human and operational resources, such as opportunities for enhancement of professional growth and quality management

6. The answer is C. (Reference: p. 82, Table 6–1)

Table 6–1. *Examples of occupational health nursing practice activities within a prevention framework*

Primary	Secondary	Tertiary
Immunizations	Health assessment and surveillance	Work hardening
Wellness programs	Preplacement/periodic examinations	Rehabilitation
Nutrition education	Screening programs, e.g., high blood pressure, mammography	Disability management
Exercise/fitness programs		

CHAPTER 7 ANSWERS

1. The answer is D. (Reference: p. 85)

IMEs are examinations performed by a physician not involved in the person's care for the purpose of clarifying medical and job issues. Key issues associated with an IME differ from clinical consultations in role and focus (Table 7–1). Occupational medicine physicians are often the most appropriate specialists to evaluate work-related injuries and other disability cases to determine whether work-site accommodations may be necessary for certain medical disorders.

2. The answer is A. (Reference: p. 86)

Clinical impressions include not only the primary illness or injury, but also other conditions that need further evaluation. It is useful to prepare a problem list of clinical diagnoses, particularly other pertinent conditions that contribute to the patient's functional status. It is helpful to present the problem list in relative order of significance, and to number each problem.

Pain, pathology, impairment, residual functional capacity, and disability are separate concepts. Pain, especially chronic pain, may not be associated with significant physical pathology (Loesser, 1991; Spektor, 1990). Pathology may be present without symptoms or dysfunction. Impairment is a measurable decrement in some physiologic function, whereas disability considers not only the physical or mental impairment but also the social, psychological, or vocational factors associated with a person's ability to work (Ryley et al., 1988; Vasudevan, 1991). Functional limitations are manifestations of impairment (Vasudevan, 1991). Factors relating to each of these issues should be identified in the problem list.

3. The answer is C. (Reference: p. 87)

Causation is a critical issue in work-related and liability cases. A work-related problem is defined as one that "arose out of and during the course of employment" (Larson, 1982). With an acute injury such as a fracture, this determination may be simple. In many workers' compensation cases, however, the process is far more complex, particularly with preexisting, chronic conditions and environmental exposures.

The physician must establish causation to a reasonable degree of medical probability, which implies that it is more probable than not (i.e., there is more than a 50% probability) that a certain condition arose out of or in the course of work duties. Possibility implies less than 50% likelihood. Stating that a problem is work related implies that, based on the available information, to a reasonable degree of medical certainty, work activities caused the problem. States may vary in the definition of causation, particularly for cumulative trauma disorders and preexisting conditions.

Apportionment refers to the extent to which a problem is caused by various factors. For example, a worker may have sustained an injury with one employer, then returned

Table 7–1. *Key issues in an independent medical evaluation (IME)*

Diagnoses
Causal relationship
Prognosis
Maximum medical improvement
Permanent impairment
Work capacity
Disability
Appropriateness of care
Recommendations

to work and sustained a similar injury with another employer. In reviewing the case, it may be necessary to apportion current dysfunction between the two parties. It also may be necessary to apportion responsibility between work-related and non–work-related conditions. This process depends largely on judgment, since the science supporting apportionment is in its infancy.

Different definitions of causation may exist for physical and mental conditions; for example, a mental condition may be attributed to work activities only if the factors associated with the illness were unique.

4. The answer is A. (Reference: p. 89)

Maximal medical improvement is a phrase used to indicate when further recovery and restoration of function can no longer be anticipated to a reasonable degree of medical probability. This assessment implies that a condition is permanent and static. Considerations include whether the current or proposed treatment will result in functional improvement, if surgery has occurred recently, and whether enough time has passed for the process to be stable.

5. The answer is C. (Reference: p. 89)

Impairment is "the loss of, the loss of use of, or a derangement of any body part, system or function." Disability is "the limiting loss of the capacity to meet personal, social, or occupational demands, or to meet statutory or regulatory requirements."

Impairment is a measurable decrement in health status evaluated by medical means; disability is the gap between what a person can do and what he or she needs to do, partly because of a diminished health status. Disability is assessed by the consideration of nonmedical issues, such as the person's educational and vocational skills, experience, age, and, in workers' compensation cases, potential for future loss of wages. Assessing education, vocation, and potential for future loss of wages is not a skill most physicians possess, and thus the medical role usually is limited to evaluating impairment, not disability (Babitsky and Sewall, 1992).

What does impairment reflect? An erroneous impression is to think that an evaluation of impairment is indicative of a person's ability or inability to do a task or set of tasks relating to work. Rather, an impairment evaluation is based on activities of daily living. Note that specific tasks of employment are not considered activities of daily living for the purposes of an impairment evaluation.

6. The answer is C. (Reference: pp. 92–96)

It is important to review the medical records before the evaluation and to read correspondence from the client, so that the evaluation can be structured to answer specific questions. The examinee may be asked to complete a questionnaire before the evaluation, to facilitate the interview. Pain and functional inventories are particularly helpful in identifying behavioral and psychological components related to an illness or injury.

At the beginning of the visit, the physician should explain the nature of the evaluation and that an independent evaluation will be conducted, but that no treatment will be performed. There is no patient–physician relationship, and a report will be sent to the requesting client.

The history, organized in sections, usually commences with a detailed review of the *injury* or illness, including the reported mechanism, symptoms at the time, and events immediately thereafter.

The history includes relevant *preexisting conditions* and prior injuries. The patient's baseline is established to determine the framework for examining the effect of the referenced condition.

The *chronology* of events from the time of injury through the present is examined.

The *current status* is explored in detail, with attention directed to the examinee's primary concern.

The person's perceived *functional status* is documented to clarify both work capacity and behavioral issues.

The complete medical history concludes with a traditional past medical history that notes medical and surgical procedures, medications and allergies, review of systems, and family history.

Radiographic films brought by the examinee (or supplied by the client) are reviewed at the visit. The findings are compared with those of the reviewing radiologist. Additional studies may be recommended to the referring source; however, they should not be obtained without approval from the referral source to avoid conflicts regarding fiscal responsibilities for the testing.

7. The answer is B. (Reference: pp. 91, 92)

Functional performance assessments are more accurate determinations of ability, if the assessment is valid and reliable and relates to particular jobs. Caution should be exercised because various methodologies are available. A structured protocol is essential. It is customary to express work capacity following parameters in the *Dictionary of Occupational Titles,* U.S. Department of Labor, which are based primarily on lifting requirements.

The examining physician should estimate capacities as carefully as possible, including the number of hours of work per day, based on endurance and tolerance for sitting, standing, and walking. Estimates of lifting and carrying capabilities are noted for specific frequencies. Guidelines should be provided for the frequency and duration of tasks such as bending, crouching, squatting, pushing/pulling, climbing stairs, climbing ladders, reaching above shoulder level, lifting above shoulder level, balancing, and working on uneven ground or at heights.

These capacities are compared with the functional requirements of the job, obtained from job descriptions, videotapes, or direct observations. The physician must advise in consideration of the Americans with Disabilities Act, and avoid arbitrary restrictions that do not meet the criteria of a direct threat. Specific assessments of work capacity based only on a clinical evaluation may be difficult.

CHAPTER 8 ANSWERS

1. The answer is A. (Reference: pp. 106, 107)

Opportunities for physicians to work closely with the business community are virtually limitless in the 1990s.

Close associations with employers are becoming a paramount positioning strategy for both physicians and medical centers as the private sector assumes greater influence in health care funding and medical service delivery.

Health care delivery is moving toward managed competition, with greater emphasis on employer responsibility.

Several significant changes have occurred in the regulatory environment that affect occupational medical practice. The deregulatory fervor of the 1980s has been overshadowed by public health regulation, especially enforcement activities. Recent initiatives include the Americans with Disabilities Act, the Drug-Free Workplace Act, and the OSHA Blood-Borne Pathogens Standard. As regulatory reforms continue in both scope and enforcement, employers need even more counsel by qualified occupational medicine practitioners.

Health care cost control is a major motivator for employers to establish partnerships with providers, especially physicians, the essential ingredients for addressing the complex occupational and environmental health issues facing business today.

Perhaps the most profound change in the practice of medicine is the decline of fee-for-service reimbursement in favor of a variety of managed care arrangements.

Reimbursement for workers' compensation–related medical care is becoming more tightly controlled through the use of nurse managers and other gatekeepers who encourage return to work and scrutinize the need for additional diagnostic testing. Workers' compensation reform will ultimately force both providers and employers to become more prevention oriented.

2. The answer is D. (Reference: p. 108)

The practice of medicine in the United States appears poised for a significant change in which physicians are evaluated on both their ability to address broad community health care concerns and their clinical skills. Accordingly, prevention is likely to assume a more pronounced role, both in reducing workplace risk factors and in using the workplace as a forum for health education. At its best, occupational medicine is a preventive discipline, as evidenced by its specialty oversight by the American Board of Preventive Medicine.

The successful occupational physician of the 1990s will be adept at organizational dynamics, consumer education, entrepreneurship, and marketing, along with the clinical practice of medicine. Occupational medicine necessitates the ability to work as part of a team, deal with multiple constituencies (e.g., employers, workers, insurance carriers), and show leadership.

The traditional physician-hospital relationship is also changing. Both groups are recognizing that collaborative arrangements may be the best way to address the broad opportunities in ambulatory care.

Hospitals and physicians who work as partners can be significant players in a competitive market (Reece and Coombes, 1993).

3. The answer is C. (Reference: p. 109)

In the past, injury care and other occupational health-related services were loosely provided out of hospital emergency departments. Today, injury care is bundled with other health-related services to create a defined product line.

Furthermore, hospital-affiliated programs have matured and are expanding services to include screening, education, and rehabilitation services along with injury management and other core services. A hospital base provides several competitive advantages:

Hospitals possess a breadth of services to offer a comprehensive approach in one setting.
Hospitals typically have the financial resources to withstand a development period that may last 12 to 18 months.
Hospitals can profit from existing personnel in management, finance, and marketing to offer immediate support for a program.

The physician/medical director is a critical part of the hospital-affiliated program team. Given the chronic undersupply of trained occupational medicine physicians, compensation and negotiation leverage is favorable for the physician. Compensation for medical directors is becoming more creative and ranges from direct salary, to salary plus incentive, to salary plus fee for service.

4. The answer is D. (Reference: p. 109)

Freestanding occupational health clinics with no formal ties to a hospital are also growing rapidly. Such clinics can include ambulatory care in addition to occupational medicine. Many successful clinics are large and multispecialty while others may involve only a few physicians or a single practitioner.

The freestanding occupational health clinic is likely to provide the physician with greater autonomy; it also gives employers an impression of greater efficiency, easier access, and less cost than services provided by hospitals. Many primary care physicians have sought to increase their patient base by offering occupational medicine services as an adjunct to an existing primary care practice.

As employers become more prudent users of occupational health services, physicians will need to broaden their services and become better acquainted with the workplace. The era of the freestanding injury care mill that lacked an appreciation of the gamut of occupational health responsibilities is beginning to slip away.

5. The answer is B. (Reference: p. 110)

Opportunities to work directly with employers are considerable, including more than one employer on a part-time basis. The more compelling opportunity, however, may be to develop a relatively narrow niche of expertise and provide replicable services to large numbers of organizations. Examples of services include advice related to medical surveillance, training, health policy, program development, and regulatory compliance. Cost-containment activities such as workers' compensation loss control (McCunney and Barbanel, 1993) and managed care are increasingly discussed with occupational medicine consultants.

6. The answer is D. (Reference: pp. 110, 111)

In a dynamic field replete with opportunity, a physician may wonder where to start. There are seven key elements to developing a profile that will allow the physician to succeed and be instrumental when working with the business community to prevent and manage work-related ailments:

1. Gain a basic foundation in occupational medicine.
2. Address the range of occupational medicine.
3. Remain abreast of regulatory measures.
4. Address interventions in terms of health care cost containment.
5. Be an educator.
6. Be prepared to play multiple roles.
7. Commit to professional and aggressive marketing.

CHAPTER 9 ANSWERS

1. The answer is B. (Reference: p. 116)

There are six major situations in which drug testing is performed at the work site:

Preemployment/preplacement
Periodic
Postaccident/incident
Reasonable cause/reasonable suspicion
Return to duty and follow-up
Random

2. The answer is A. (Reference: pp. 117, 118)

Urine collection is particularly crucial because so many errors occur here. It is vitally important that the urine collection process treat each person with respect and allow the maximum reasonable privacy, while minimizing the opportunity to substitute or adulterate urine specimens. Attention to detail in completing paperwork is also essential. Most positive drug tests that are invalidated are due to improper urine collection or documentation.

There are three ways to conduct urine collection. In private collection, the donor provides a specimen in a separate room with complete privacy. In monitored collection, the urine collection is conducted in a public restroom or other facility that offers partial privacy, for example, inside a stall with partitions that block direct view. A licensed health professional of either gender may monitor urine collection; a nonmedically licensed collector must be the same gender as the donor. The third form of collection is under direct observation of the urine exiting the urinary meatus—so-called witnessed collection. Collection site personnel must be the same gender as the donor when a collection is conducted under direct supervision.

Following collection, the collector and the donor should keep the sample in constant view until it is sealed and labeled. The collector places a tamper-proof seal on the specimen bottle's cap and down the sides of the bottle, together with an identification label showing the date and specimen identification number. The tested individual must initial the label to certify that it is the specimen collected from him or her.

If an employer has requested both a federally mandated drug test for the NIDA-5 and a test for additional drugs, separate specimens must be collected (separate urine voids into separate containers) for the federally mandated test and for the additional drugs. It is unacceptable to pour any remaining urine from the void for the federally mandated test into another container for additional drug testing. Separate custody and control forms must be used for each specimen.

3. The answer is D. (Reference: pp. 122, 123, 125)

Many prescription and over-the-counter (OTC) drugs can cause positive test results. Verification of legitimate medical explanations for positive tests often requires clinical judgment. For example, tetrahydrocannabinol, the active ingredient of marijuana, is used as an antinausea agent for cancer patients under the prescription name Marinol. Although inhalation of sidestream marijuana smoke is offered as an explanation for a positive test result, toxicology studies have not confirmed this explanation as feasible. Cocaine is used in ear-nose-throat (ENT), ophthalmology, and surgical procedures, such as injection of TAC (tetracaine, adrenaline, and cocaine) for suturing skin lacerations. Because extremely high doses of ephedrine or l-methamphetamine (e.g., Vicks Inhaler) can cause a positive immunoassay screening, the MRO should request d- and l-isomer isolation on confirmed methamphetamine specimens with a level over 10,000 ng/ml. Ingestion of poppy seeds can cause high levels of urine opiates. The federal regulations require that verification of an opiate test as positive requires clinical confirmation of opiate abuse, or the identification of the heroin metabolite monoacetylmorphine (6-MAM). Clinical signs include medical history, physical findings, or behavior fitting DSM-III (*Diagnostic and Statistical Manual of Mental Disorders,* 3rd ed.). Definitions of opiate abuse ascertained by a trained medical professional (DSM-III, 1982). Medical review officers must determine whether quantitative levels are compatible with prescription drug use.

Another issue in MRO judgment involves the use of medication prescribed for one's spouse, child, or other relative or acquaintance. DOT recommends that these be verified as positive, that is, representing unauthorized use of controlled substances. Unless this issue is specifically addressed in company policy, consideration of whether spousal use is legitimate or unauthorized drug use remains an MRO judgment. It is best to resolve this issue in advance through consultation with the employer. This is also true regarding use of a dated prescription issued to the individual tested. It is important for the MRO to document evidence provided as substantiation of authorized drug use.

4. The answer is E. (Reference: p. 126)

Because of concerns about quality of MRO services, federal officials urged establishment of voluntary MRO credentialing and certification within the private sectors. Although MRO certification is not required by current federal regulations, physicians seeking to demonstrate their competence in a competitive marketplace and a litigious environment have shown strong interest in MRO credentialing. The Medical Review Officer Certification Council (MROCC) was established in 1992 by ACOEM. MROCC eligibility requires at least 12 hours of approved MRO training, followed by a rigorous certifying examination (Medical Review Officer Certification Council). Certificates are valid for 5 years.

5. The answer is A. (Reference: p. 117)

Federal regulations contain detailed procedures for urine collection, completion of custody and control forms, analysis by laboratories certified by the National Institute on Drug Abuse (NIDA) for only five specified illicit drugs (amphetamines, cocaine, marijuana, opiates, and phencyclidine—the NIDA-5), and mandatory reporting of all results to an MRO for review and interpretation before reporting to the employer.

6. The answer is A. (Reference: pp. 130, 131)

The following features should be included in any program for the screening of employees and prospective employees for drugs:

1. A written company policy and procedure concerning drug use and screening for the presence of drugs should exist and be applied impartially.
2. The reason for any requirement for screening for drugs should be clearly documented. Such reasons might involve safety for the individual, other employees, or the public; security needs; or requirements related to job performance.
3. Affected employees and applicants should be informed in advance about the company's policy concerning drug use and screening. They should be made aware of their right to refuse such screening and the consequences of such refusal to their employment.
4. Where special safety or security needs justify testing for drugs on an unannounced and possibly random basis, employees should be made aware in advance that this will be done from time to time. Care should be taken to assure that such tests are done in a uniform and impartial manner for all employees in the affected group(s).
5. Written consent for screening and for communication of results to the employer should be obtained from each individual prior to screening.

6. Collection, transportation, and analysis of the specimens and the reporting of the results should meet stringent legal, technical, and ethical requirements. The process should be under the supervision of a licensed physician.

7. A licensed physician who is qualified as a medical review officer should evaluate positive results before a report is made to the employer.

8. The affected employee or applicant should be advised of positive results by the physician and have the opportunity for explanation and discussion prior to the reporting of results to the employer, if feasible.

9. The employee or applicant having indication of a drug abuse problem should be advised concerning appropriate treatment resources.

10. Any report to the employer should provide only the information needed for work placement purposes or as required by government regulations.

7. The answer is D. (Reference: p. 125)

Tests must be conducted using evidential grade breath testing devices approved by the National Highway Transportation Safety Administration (NHTSA). Confirmation tests must provide a permanent record of results and identification of the individual tested (e.g., a printed result of sequentially numbered tests), be capable of testing blank air samples, and discriminate between alcohol and acetone, which can be produced by diabetics in ketoacidosis. Both initial screening and confirmation tests will be required, with a 15-minute wait between tests. The lower of the two results determines the consequence. Testing must be conducted by a trained, certified breath alcohol technician (BAT) who has demonstrated proficiency in a NHTSA-approved course.

Employees with alcohol concentrations of 0.04 or greater will be removed from safety-sensitive duty. Return to work will be permitted only after evaluation and rehabilitation, if indicated, as well as follow-up testing.

CHAPTER 10 ANSWERS

1. The answer is B. (Reference: pp. 132, 133)

Medical organizations may pursue accreditation for a variety of reasons. In some cases, the sole motivation may be to improve operations and quality of care. Here, the value of accreditation will depend on several elements: first, the relevance of the standards to the specific medical organization; second, the emphasis of the standards on assuring and improving quality of care; third, the amount of consultative assistance provided by the accreditation organization in the process of performing the audit. In other cases, the organization's primary goal may be financial: assuring reimbursement, expanding market shares, or reducing insurance premiums. Here, the value of accreditation depends on the credibility and prestige of the accrediting body, specifically whether accreditation assures payment or financial gain. Based on experience with hospitals, accreditation only becomes widespread when it is linked to reimbursement.

AAAHC is a nonprofit corporation whose goal is to assist ambulatory health care organizations in providing high-quality care in the most efficient and economically sound manner possible. AAAHC achieves its goal through a voluntary, peer-based accreditation program that is focused on education and counseling.

The organization was founded in 1979, though its charter members have been involved in accreditation issues since the mid-1960s. The development of AAAHC was prompted by a reorganization of the Joint Commission for the Accreditation of Hospitals (now the Joint Commission on Accreditation of Healthcare Organizations). The reorganization eliminated the Council for Ambulatory Health Care and replaced it with technical and consulting services. Believing that this was inadequate, several organizations that were involved with the Joint Commission joined together to form AAAHC.

There are 22 individual standards, which are divided into two groups: core and adjunct. Core standards apply to all organizations and address issues common to ambulatory health care delivery, such as administration, facilities, and records. Adjunct standards address specific services or activities and only apply if the organization is active in these areas. One of the adjunct standards is occupational health services.

2. The answer is A. (Reference: pp. 133, 134)

AAAHC's goal is to provide quality accreditation services to a wide variety of ambulatory health care organizations. This goal is reflected in the eligibility requirements for accreditation surveys, which are summarized as follows: The organization's primary activity must be provision of health services and it must have been in operation for at least 6 months. Either the organization or its parent organization must be a formally organized, legal entity. If required, the organization must be licensed to provide services and be in compliance with appropriate regulations. For occupational health services, medical care must be under the direction or supervision of a physician(s). The health care organization must also share facilities, equipment, and patient care records among its members providing patient care.

3. The answer is D. (Reference: pp. 134, 135)

The first step of the self-assessment process is creation of a committee or team. Collectively, the members of this team should be knowledgeable about all aspects of the organization's operations, be capable of implementing change, and be committed to the process of self-assessment and accreditation. Once the committee is formed, it identifies a chairperson and divides primary responsibilities for the standards among its members. These individuals enlist the support of other organization members, begin the process of assessment, and plan for needed changes. One of the goals at this step of the process is to involve as much of the organization as possible. Ultimately, everyone will be affected by the accreditation process. Through regular meetings, the team creates a timetable for the project and monitors progress.

The self-assessment process may take months to years depending on the status of the organization.

Once the self-assessment is completed, the organization obtains, completes, and submits the Presurvey Questionnaire.

The survey consists of an extensive on-site evaluation of the organization's policies, procedures, and operations.

A primary goal of the surveyors is to determine if the organization is in compliance with the intent of the standards.

A second goal of the surveyors is to educate and provide consultation to the organization.

Accreditation can be granted for either 1 or 3 years. AAAHC can also decide to defer accreditation if there are deficiencies that are likely to be corrected within 6 months. A third option is to register the survey as a consultation, which occurs if AAAHC finds that the standards are not appropriate for the facility. Lastly, AAAHC may deny accreditation. There is a formal policy for appeals and the organization can apply for reevaluation immediately.

4. The answer is E. (Reference: pp. 135, 136)

The following eight topics constitute AAAHC's core standards. All organizations must be in compliance with these standards: (1) patient rights, (2) governance, (3) administration, (4) quality of care, (5) quality assurance, (6) clinical records, (7) professional improvement, and (8) facilities and environment.

5. The answer is B. (Reference: pp. 136, 137)

The most pertinent of the adjunct standards is occupational health services. This set of criteria was developed by ACOEM and adopted by AAAHC. The opening statement sets the goals of occupational health services as assuring a safe and healthy workplace through the recognition, evaluation, and control of illness and injury in or from the workplace. The organization must also meet the needs of the employees.

The standard itself contains 12 points, which are summarized as follows:

1. Services must be in compliance with all pertinent regulations including the Occupational Safety and Health Act and workers' compensation laws. This point was written before the enactment of the Americans with Disabilities Act, which should also be addressed.
2. Individuals providing services must be appropriately trained, have necessary skills, and be knowledgeable about the work environment and the specific risks for the individual patient.
3. Individuals must have access to reference materials and an occupational health physician.
4. Continuing education in occupational health is specifically required.
5. Medical management includes consideration of the relationship of the patient's condition to work, the effect of the condition on fitness for duty, and consideration of disability status.
6. Medical care should strive to minimize disability and restore function as soon as possible.
7. If the patient is off work, the health care provider should consider issues regarding his or her safe return to work. This assessment includes the prognosis for functional improvement, the potential hazards that may interfere with a return to work, and ways to reduce these hazards.

8. Preplacement examinations must consider both the patient's medical status and the work demands. Therefore, both the employee and health provider must know the essential job functions and workplace conditions. All findings and recommendations should be reviewed with the employee; the employer should be informed of the recommendations.

9. Medical surveillance examinations should be appropriately timed to identify adverse health effects of workplace exposures. Employees should be informed of findings and the relationship of these to work. The employers should be advised of any adverse health effects from work exposures and any recommendations regarding risk reduction. In addition, the services should educate the employee about the potential hazards of their workplace and about methods to reduce the risk. This role includes consideration of lifestyle habits, if the habits may affect the risk of workplace exposures.

10. Information that does not relate to the employee's ability to safely perform the job must be handled as confidential and only be released with proper consent, and only if there is a need to know.

11. The organization's records management system must be able to report health surveillance data and any other statutory requirements.

12. If the occupational medicine (OM) service is a subunit within a larger organization, the organization's management must demonstrate that it understands and supports the services provided.

6. The answer is A. (Reference: pp. 137, 138)

Deficiencies in medical records are among the most common problems seen in surveys. The clinical record work sheet in the Handbook provides 16 specific areas that are used to judge care and medical records. The standard indicates that records must be legible, accurate, current, and accessible, and have a common format. All information, including test reports, dictated notes, and hospitalization records, must be reviewed. In addition, the chart must clearly note allergies. Problems can arise in any of these areas, but a common problem is failing to adequately document the patient encounter.

The medical record is the most common source of information about patient care. It is used by all accrediting bodies including the AAAHC. To evaluate care, the medical records must provide sufficient detail so that an outside reviewer can (1) determine the patient's primary complaint, (2) independently confirm the patient's diagnosis based on reported findings, (3) confirm that the treatment was appropriate and necessary, and (4) confirm that the patient's care was appropriate over time. Records must be complete and legible.

7. The answer is D. (Reference: p. 139)

Standards of care are important elements of quality assurance programs; however, some physicians are reluctant to participate in any program that may develop such standards. The rationale for their concern varies. In some cases, physicians believe that guidelines will substitute cookbook medicine for clinical judgment. Alternatively they may be concerned that the process is attempting to identify individuals for punitive measures. Neither is true. Practice guidelines attempt to create a template for the best quality care for patients. Clinical judgment is required in developing the guidelines, which may need to be modified and applied to specific patients.

Developing guidelines relies on aggregate data that summarize the experience with many patients. They do not rely on data from a single physician. Furthermore, guideline development focuses on processes, not on individuals.

Section 2

Occupational Pulmonary Disease

OBJECTIVES

- List four major categories of occupational lung disorders
- Cite differences between latency in acute and chronic occupational lung disease
- Explain the range of tests used for the evaluation of occupational lung disease
- State the contributions of the B-reader
- Explain complications that may develop from toxic exposure to the respiratory tract

OUTLINE

I. Diagnosis
    A. Patient Evaluation
        1. History
        2. Physical Examination
    B. Laboratory Evaluation
        1. Chest X-ray
        2. Lung Function Tests
            Figure 11–1. Volume-time and flow volume curves
        3. Airway Challenge Testing
        4. Bronchoscopy and Bronchoalveolar Lavage
        5. Immunologic Tests
    C. Formulating a Diagnosis
II. Common Occupational Pulmonary Disorders
    A. The Pneumoconioses
        1. Silicosis
        2. Coal Worker's Pneumoconiosis
        3. Asbestosis
        4. Other Pneumoconioses
    B. Irritant Lung Reactions
        Table 11–1. Characteristics of some common irritant gases and fumes

Table 11–2. Principles for the management of acute pulmonary
effects from inhaling irritant gases, fumes, and aerosols.
C. Occupational Asthma
Table 11–3. Agents that cause occupational asthma
D. Hypersensitivity Pneumonitis (Extrinsic Allergic Alveolitis)
Table 11–4. Some causes of extrinsic allergic alveolitis
III. Prevention
Table 11–5. OSHA standards for occupational respiratory hazards
IV. References

KEY POINTS

- An occupational lung disorder is an acute or chronic lung condition that arises, at least partly, from the inhalation of an airborne agent in the workplace. Occupational lung disorders include diseases caused solely by workplace exposures, as well as conditions such as asthma that may predate workplace exposures but are exacerbated by them.
- Occupational lung disorders fall into four major categories: pneumoconioses or "dust-related" disease, irritant reactions, asthmatic responses, and hypersensitivity reactions.
- The diagnosis of occupational lung disease can only be made if a physician is in the habit of asking a patient about his or her work. Acute lung disorders, such as irritant or hypersensitivity reactions, are more likely to be related to workplace exposures at the time symptoms first appear. Some diseases that cause chronic progressive disability (such as advanced silicosis, asbestosis, or coal worker's pneumoconiosis) generally have a period of at least 10 years of exposure to the relevant dust; even with 10 years of exposure, it may be 20 or more years from first exposure before evidence of a pneumoconiosis appears.
- Information that other workers in the same area or doing similar jobs were affected similarly is supportive of a work-related etiology.
- A chest x-ray and spirometry are essential to the assessment of occupational lung disease. When any of the pneumoconioses, asbestos-related pleural disease, or berylliosis is suspected, the chest films should be read according to the classification that has been developed by the International Labor Office (ILO) of the World Health Organization based on the nature, size, and extent of opacities. Only certain radiologists and physicians are certified to read films according to this classification. These physicians are termed B-readers.
- Lung function tests can be used to assign respiratory impairment in terms of abnormal spirometry. By convention, ventilatory abnormalities are described either as being obstructive (defined as an abnormally decreased forced expiratory volume in 1 second (FEV_1) and decreased FEV_1/forced vital capacity (FVC) ratio) or restrictive (an abnormally decreased FVC with well-preserved FEV_1/FVC ratio).
- Bronchial provocation tests are particularly useful when assessing patients with possible occupational asthma. Nonspecific airway challenge tests determine whether an individual's airways are unusually "reactive" to a nonspecific bronchoconstrictor stimulus, such as methacholine. Specific airways provocation tests involve exposure of the subject to the agent(s) thought to cause asthma.
- Other studies that may be helpful include fiberoptic bronchoscopy and brushings, transbronchial biopsy, and bronchoalveolar lavage.
- Immune-mediated occupational lung disorders include asthma and "extrinsic allergic alveolitis." Specific immunoglobulin E (IgE) has been demonstrated for several causes of occupational asthma, and antibodies may be detected by the radioallergosorbent test (RAST). Immune testing seems to have the greatest predictive value in chronic beryllium disease.

- Silicosis is the most common pneumoconiosis worldwide. People who work in mines or are involved in blasting and drilling operations are at risk of exposure to silica. Other high-risk groups include sandblasters and foundry workers.
- A definite increase in the risk of pulmonary tuberculosis is attributed to silica exposure. A variant of silicosis occurs in patients who have rheumatoid arthritis or circulating rheumatoid factor; these patients can develop necrobiotic nodules several centimeters in diameter that frequently cavitate and become infected (Caplan's syndrome).
- Asbestosis is a form of lung fibrosis of the "usual interstitial type" that results from the inhalation of asbestos fibers. The term *asbestosis* refers only to this type of parenchymal lung disease and excludes pleural thickening or fibrosis that may accompany the parenchymal lesions. Asbestos bodies (or ferruginous bodies) are composed of an asbestos fiber that has been subjected to attack by alveolar macrophages with the resulting deposition of proteinaceous materials and iron on the surface of the fiber.
- Many gases, fumes, and aerosols are directly toxic to the respiratory tract by causing acute inflammation of the respiratory mucosa and lung parenchyma. The principal sites in the respiratory tract where different agents have the greatest effect are determined by their water solubility and particle size. Highly soluble agents dissolve readily in the upper respiratory tract and airways; less-soluble agents exert their main effects in the peripheral, small airways and in the lung parenchyma. Pleural larger than 10 μm in diameter tend to settle in the upper respiratory tract; those 3 to 10 μm settle mainly in the airways; those smaller than 3 μm deposit mainly in the lung parenchyma and small airways.
- Exposures to high air concentrations of water-soluble agents cause extensive inflammatory changes throughout the respiratory tract. In severe cases, this amounts to a chemical burn of the respiratory mucosa and is a medical emergency. Two principal problems that may result are laryngeal edema and severe lung edema, which may require assisted ventilation and oxygen. The serious sequel of toxic irritants are not always apparent at the time of exposure, but may develop 24 to 48 hours later. Long-term complications of toxic edema may include lung fibrosis and occasionally bronchiolitis obliterans.
- Reactive airways dysfunction syndrome (RADS) may follow acute exposures to lung irritants. Individuals may develop the onset of asthma or experience the return of asthma after many years.
- Occupational asthma may be diagnosed by (1) demonstrating that an individual has asthma (using lung spirometry or, if baseline lung function is normal, by showing that the individual has nonspecific airway hyperactivity) and (2) demonstrating a causal link between workplace exposure and alterations in lung function. Bronchial challenge in the laboratory or in the work site with the agent(s) of interest may be useful. Specific bronchial provocation tests are best performed by experienced personnel in a laboratory where the nature of the exposure can be controlled and where urgent treatment can be administered promptly for an acute severe reaction. Once a diagnosis of occupational asthma is established, prompt job transfer is necessary to an area of no exposure.
- Farmer's lung is a type of hypersensitivity (type III) pneumonitis that resembles recurrent pneumonia. It is most commonly due to the bacteria *Micropolyspora faeni* and various fungi, such as thermophilic actinomyces species.

QUESTIONS

*1. Irritant lung reactions are **least** likely to:*

A. depend on water solubility.
B. depend on particle size.

   C. lead to fibrosis.
   D. lead to reactive airways dysfunction syndrome.
   E. depend on particle shape.

2. *Which statement is **incorrect** regarding hypersensitivity pneumonitis?*

   A. It results from inhalation of organic antigenic dusts.
   B. It has findings that suggest infectious disease (fever, chills, increased white count).
   C. It is an immune disease mediated by IgG antigen complexes.
   D. It is treated with antibiotics and bronchodilators.
   E. Chronic exposure may lead to fibrosis.

3. *Respiratory disease may be categorized as obstructive or restrictive based on spirometric testing. Typically, an obstructive pattern would be:*

   A. abnormally decreased FVC with normal FEV_1/FVC ratio.
   B. abnormally decreased FEV_1 with decreased FEV_1/FVC ratio.
   C. abnormally decreased FVC and FEV_1 with mild increase in FEV_1/FVC ratio.
   D. only A and B above.
   E. none of the above.

4. *Pneumoconioses are dust inhalation diseases that are characterized by chest x-ray abnormalities in all cases and clinical respiratory impairment in most cases. Which one of the following has the **least** clinical impairment?*

   A. asbestosis
   B. silicosis
   C. stannosis
   D. talcosis
   E. coal worker's pneumoconiosis

5. *Which of the following is **incorrect** regarding occupational asthma?*

   A. Low molecular weight agents may precipitate occupational asthma.
   B. Onset of symptoms may be abrupt and in the workplace.
   C. High molecular weight agents may precipitate occupational asthma.
   D. Onset may be delayed for several hours after exposure.
   E. Responsible agents always exceed PELs.

12

Musculoskeletal Disorders

OBJECTIVES

- List the importance of acute back injuries from workplace exposure
- Enumerate the essentials of the evaluation of low back pain
- List therapeutic steps after low back injury
- Distinguish between acute and chronic low back pain
- State important issues in the prevention of back injuries
- List various types of cumulative trauma disorders that involve the upper extremity

OUTLINE

I. Rates of Occupational Injuries
II. Back Disorders

  A. Acute Back Injuries
  B. The Diagnosis of Low Back Pain

    1. History

      Table 12–1. Back compensation claims by occupation

    2. Physical Examination
    3. Diagnostic Imaging
    4. Acute Management of Low Back Pain
    5. Medical Follow-Up of Low Back Injury

  C. Chronic Back Disorders

    1. History
    2. Laboratory Testing

      Table 12–2. Causes of low back pain

    3. Electromyography/Nerve Conduction Velocity (EMG/NCV)

      Table 12–3. Nonorganic physical signs in low back pain

    4. Treatment
    5. Rehabilitation and Return to Work Status

      Table 12–4. Laboratory tests of potential value in assessing chronic back pain

  D. Prevention of Back Injuries

   1. Proper Selection and Placement
   2. Maintenance of a Healthy Back
  III. Shoulder Disorders
  IV. Knee Injuries
   V. Cumulative Trauma Disorders
   A. Carpal Tunnel Syndrome
    1. History
    2. Physical Examination
    3. Electromyography/Nerve Conduction Velocity
    4. Treatment
   B. Wrist Tendinitis
   C. Hand-Arm Vibration Syndrome
   D. Epicondylitis
   E. Other Nerve Entrapment Syndromes
  VI. Neck Injuries
  VII. References

KEY POINTS

- Occupational back pain is the most common musculoskeletal complaint in the workplace. Risk factors for low back pain include heavy repetitive lifting, pushing, and pulling as well as exposure to industrial and vehicular vibration. In addition, other psychosocial risk factors include previous back injury claims, job dissatisfaction, poor ratings from supervisors, repetitive boring tasks, younger age, shorter duration of employment, smoking, and a history of non–back injury claims.
- Most low back pain problems are diagnosed and treated by primary care physicians.
- Low back pain may be due to a variety of causes, including (1) musculoligamentous injuries; (2) vertebral fractures; (3) degenerative changes; (4) spinal stenosis; (5) anatomic anomalies, such as spondylolisthesis; (6) herniated intervertebral disks; (7) systemic diseases such as cancer, spinal infections, and ankylosing spondylitis; and (8) visceral diseases unrelated to the spine.
- The cornerstones of treatment for low back pain arising from a work-related episode are rest and symptomatic relief of discomfort.
- Frequent follow-up examinations, especially in the early phase of an injury, are advisable.
- Chronic back pain refers to back pain that has been present for over 6 weeks and that has not responded to conservative measures.
- An effective program for prevention of back injuries depends on proper selection and placement of employees, appropriate job design, maintenance of health through education, and physical fitness.
- Routine lumbosacral spine films have failed to be effective in the identification of individuals predisposed to back injury.
- A variety of injuries to the shoulder or knee are common in the occupational setting.
- Cumulative trauma disorders (also known as repetitive motion injuries) are thought to be due to repetitive performance of a similar task, and primarily affect the upper extremities.
- Carpal tunnel syndrome is due to the compression of the median nerve as it traverses the carpal tunnel in the wrist.
- The NIOSH criteria for diagnosis include (1) symptoms suggestive of carpal tunnel syndrome; (2) objective findings, which can include either a positive Tinel's or Phalen's sign, decreased sensation in the distribution of the median nerve, or abnormal electrodiagnostic findings of the median nerve across the carpal tunnel; and (3) evidence of work-relatedness.

- The hand-arm vibration syndrome, formerly known as vibration white finger, is thought to be due to arterial spasm (similar to Raynaud's phenomenon) and muscle fatigue as a result of the vibration of a tool.
- Epicondylitis involving either the medial or lateral epicondyle of the elbow may be due to excessive stress on the muscle groups around the elbow and forearm.
- Neck injuries involving muscular strain and spasm are common in the occupational setting.

QUESTIONS

1. *Which of the following is a significant risk factor for disabling occupational back pain?*

A. Job dissatisfaction
B. Poor ratings from supervisors
C. Cigarette smoking
D. History of non–back injury claims
E. All of the above

2. *All of the following are risk factors for the development of protruded intervertebral disk* **except:**

A. frequent lifting of objects >25 lbs.
B. exposure to whole body vibration.
C. cigarette smoking.
D. physical fitness.
E. narrow lumbar vertebral canals.

3. *Plain films of the lumbosacral spine are indicated in the workup for suspicion of all of the following conditions* **except:**

A. vertebral fracture.
B. herniated intervertebral disk.
C. osteomyelitis of the lumbar spine.
D. primary or metastatic cancer of the lumbar spine.
E. none of the above.

4. *Management of musculoskeletal disease appropriately includes which of the following treatments?*

A. local ice
B. local heat
C. bed rest for 2 weeks
D. only A and B above
E. only A and C above

13

Occupational Cancers

OBJECTIVES

- Explain theories of carcinogenesis.
- Recall methods used in the identification of carcinogens.
- Review clinical settings that relate to questions about carcinogen exposure.

OUTLINE

KEY POINTS

- Carcinogens can be chemicals, physical agents (such as ionizing radiation), or biologic agents (such as viruses or aflatoxin).

- Although current knowledge of carcinogenesis remains incomplete, experimental work suggests there are two stages: initiation and promotion.
  - Initiation is an event in which an irreversible change occurs in the cell's genetic material known as the alteration of DNA.
  - Promotion consists of one or more subsequent steps when factors allow the transformed cell to develop into focal proliferation, such as a nodule, then to malignant tumor, and finally a metastasis.
- Studies of ribonucleic acid (RNA) viruses revealed that some coded for genetic sequences, when inserted into host genomes, could cause malignant transformation. These were called oncogenes. Some carcinogens can damage deoxyribonucleic acid (DNA) directly, but most require metabolic activation by enzymes.
- Latency refers to the period of time between onset of exposure to a carcinogen and the clinical detection of cancer. The latency period for hematologic malignancies is 2 to 5 years but the latency period for solid tumors is 10 to 50 years.
- *Threshold* is a term used for a safe level of exposure to a carcinogen, below which carcinogenesis does not occur. Whether thresholds exist is controversial.
- Carcinogens may be identified by epidemiologic studies, animal studies, in vitro test systems, and structure-activity relationships analysis. Epidemiologic studies are potentially the most definitive source of information on human carcinogenicity, since they are based on human exposure data.
- The International Agency for Research on Cancer (IARC) classifies chemical carcinogenicity with categories: group 1 includes chemicals and processes established as human carcinogens; group 2 includes those that are "probably" (group 2A) or "possibly" (group 2B) carcinogenic to humans; group 3 includes agents that are not classified; and group 4 includes agents that are probably not carcinogenic.
- In the event of exposure to a carcinogen, a physician should take steps to end such exposure by replacement of the carcinogen, enclosure of the process, or by the use of personal protective equipment.
- Carcinogens or their metabolites have been directly measured in biologic media, such as blood and urine, for many years. Perhaps the most direct approach to exposure measurement is to assess the "biologically effective dose" or a carcinogen at its ultimate target, DNA, by measuring DNA adducts. As a proxy, RNA adducts and protein adducts may also be studied.
- Markers of risk may emerge from advances in molecular biology. Three general categories are (1) markers of unusually high or low ability to metabolize carcinogens, (2) markers of low ability to repair damaged DNA, and (3) markers of other cancer-prone states.
- Markers of effect are increasingly available. These signal that a carcinogen has reached a target tissue and caused changes in genetic material that might predict the development of cancer. Cytogenetic abnormalities such as sister chromatid exchanges and micronuclei have been measured since the 1970s, and have been found to be elevated in many working populations, including those exposed to benzene, epichlorhydrin, styrene, vinyl chloride, asbestos, and ethylene oxide.
- The protein products of activated oncogenes can be detected using monoclonal antibodies, an approach with great promise in occupational medicine screening. These techniques are not ready for routine application yet, but may offer options in the future.
- The issue of cancer causation in an individual patient is difficult to address.

QUESTIONS

1. *Regarding the mechanism of environmental and occupational carcinogenesis, most carcinogens:*

A. act by directly damaging DNA.

B.   must be metabolically converted to active forms before damaging DNA.
C.   act as oncoproteins.
D.   are oncogene products.
E.   none of the above.

2.   *Which argument does **not** support threshold exposures in carcinogenesis?*

A.   There are known repair mechanisms that operate to correct DNA damage.
B.   Certain carcinogens are ubiquitous and even essential at low doses.
C.   There is no safe level of exposure to carcinogens.
D.   Carcinogens that act epigenetically often have reversible effects.
E.   Empiric data suggest the existence of threshold.

3.   *Which of the following are potentially the most definite source of information on human carcinogenicity?*

A.   Epidemiologic data
B.   Results of animal studies
C.   In vitro tests
D.   Quantitative structure-activity relationship analyses
E.   Molecular biologic studies (DNA adducts)

4.   *Of the chemicals and processes IARC has evaluated for carcinogenicity, approximately what proportion have been placed in group 1 (established human carcinogens)?*

A.   Less than 10%
B.   Less than 30%
C.   Less than 50%
D.   Less than 70%
E.   Less than 90%

5.   *Screening for cancers has been shown to achieve diagnosis at earlier stages, and consequently improved mortality, for which of the following occupational cancers?*

A.   Lung cancer among asbestos workers
B.   Bladder cancer among dye workers
C.   Leukemia among benzene workers
D.   Only B and C above
E.   None of the above

REFERENCE

Gonzalez FJ, Crespi CL, Gelboin HV. DNA-expressed human cytochrome P-450s: a new age of molecular toxicology and human risk assessment. *Mutat. Res.* 247:113, 1991.

14

Cardiovascular Disorders

OBJECTIVES

- Explain the impact of coronary heart disease in the workplace
- List the elements of a program for prevention of coronary heart disease
- Discuss methods used to assess work capability after a cardiac event
- Recall occupational agents that can cause or aggravate heart disease

OUTLINE

I. Prevention of Coronary Heart Disease in the Occupational Setting
    Table 14–1. Estimated prevalence of the major cardiovascular diseases (CVD; United States, 1989 estimate)
    Table 14–2. Estimated economic costs in billions of dollars of cardiovascular diseases by type of expenditure (United States, 1993 estimate)
  A. Blood Pressure
  B. Cigarette Smoking
  C. Cholesterol
    Table 14–3. Guidelines for patient referral based on cholesterol levels
  D. Physical Fitness
II. Assessing Work Capabilities Following a Major Cardiac Event
    Table 14–4. Factors involved in returning to work after a major cardiac event
  A. Clinical Assessment of Work Capabilities
    1. History/Physical Examination
    2. Exercise Electrocardiogram
      Table 14–5. Approximately metabolic cost of certain physical activities
    3. Job analysis
    4. Cardiac Rehabilitation
III. Occupational Agents that Cause or Aggravate Heart Disease
  A. Clinical Evaluation

      B. Cardiotoxic Agents
         1. Carbon Monoxide
         2. Solvents
         3. Carbon Disulfide
         4. Nitro Compounds
      C. Miscellaneous Agents
         Table 14–6. Agents associated with work-related cardiovascular disease
   IV. References

KEY POINTS

- Risk factors for coronary heart disease include cigarette smoking, hypertension, elevations of cholesterol, physical inactivity, obesity, increasing age, male gender, and family history.
- Efforts to prevent development of coronary heart disease depend on modification of some of these risk factors.
- Over 1.5 million Americans suffer a myocardial infarction (MI) each year, and approximately 190,000 patients have coronary artery bypass graft (CABG) surgery. One's ability to resume occupational activities depends on medical, social, and psychological factors. More than 80% of those who suffer a myocardial infarction or undergo CABG return to their original positions.
- A symptom-limited exercise test is considered to be the most sensitive predictor of future reinfarction and death if the test is performed within 6 weeks of the acute MI. Myocardial ischemia and left ventricular dysfunction, however, are the major determinants of both prognosis and functional capacity after an MI.
- Cardiac rehabilitation, especially prescribed physical activity, is accepted treatment for many patients. While cardiac exercise is generally safe, there are circumstances in which monitored exercise is prudent. The American College of Cardiology has suggested that telemetry be employed when the following conditions exist:
  - severely depressed left ventricular function (ejection fraction < 30%).
  - resting complex ventricular arrhythmia (Lown type 4 or 5).
  - ventricular arrhythmias appearing or increasing with exercise.
  - systolic blood pressure decreasing with exercise.
  - previous cardiac arrest.
  - after MI complicated by congestive heart failure, cardiogenic shock, or serious ventricular arrhythmias.
  - severe CAD and marked exercise-induced ischemia (ST depression >2 mm).
  - inability to self-monitor heart rate due to physical or intellectual impairment.
- A variety of occupational agents may cause or aggravate heart disease. These may include carbon monoxide, solvents, carbon disulfide, and nitro compounds. Methylene chloride has the unique property of being converted to carbon monoxide in vivo.

QUESTIONS

1. Which of the following is a major factor in the ability to return to work following CABG?

A. Age
B. Adequate relief of anginal pain
C. Education level
D. Psychological factors
E. All of the above

2. *Which of the following factors does **not** warrant telemetry during exercise?*

A. Severely depressed left ventricular function (ejection fraction <30%)
B. Systolic blood pressure increasing with exercise
C. Previous cardiac arrest
D. Resting complex ventricular arrhythmia
E. Inability to self-monitor heart rate due to physical or intellectual impairment

3. *Which of the following pairs of cardiac toxin/toxic effect is **incorrect?***

A. Solvents/cardiac dysrhythmia
B. Carbon disulfide/increased atherosclerosis
C. Nitro compounds/rebound coronary spasm
D. Carbon monoxide/myocardial ischemia
E. All are correct

4. *The Guidelines for Patient Referral from the National Cholesterol Education Program define borderline high cholesterol as*

A. LDL-cholesterol >160 mg/dl.
B. LDL-cholesterol <130 mg/dl.
C. risk factor ratio (total cholesterol/HDL cholesterol) >4.5.
D. total cholesterol >240 mg/dl.
E. total cholesterol 200–239 mg/dl.

REFERENCES

National Cholesterol Education Program. *Report on population strategies for blood cholesterol reduction.* Washington, DC: U.S. Department of Health and Human Services, 1990.

Position report on cardiac rehabilitation. Recommendations of the American College of Cardiology. *J. Am. Coll. Cardiol.* 7:451, 1986.

15

Neurotoxic Disorders

OBJECTIVES

- Explain how hazardous materials may damage the nervous system
- List factors that may modify an individual response to toxic exposure
- State the types of nervous system damage that may occur
- Discuss studies used in the evaluation of peripheral or central nerve system dysfunction
- Explain the neurologic of exposure to common toxicants

OUTLINE

I. Peripheral Nervous System and Toxic Effects
   A. Disorders of Peripheral Nerves
II. Electrodiagnostic Studies of Peripheral Nerve Function
III. Central Nervous System and Neurotoxic Effects
IV. Tests of Neurobehavioral Effects of Neurotoxicity
         Table 15–1. Neuropsychological test battery
V. Clinical Evaluation of Neurotoxic Symptoms
         Table 15–2. Diagnostic criteria for identifying neurotoxic effects
   A. Headache
   B. Chronic Toxic Encephalopathy
      1. Lead
      2. Arsenic
      3. Manganese
      4. Mercury
      5. Organic Solvents
      6. Organophosphate Insecticides
   C. Neurotoxic Parkinsonism
   D. Peripheral Neuropathy
      1. Lead
      2. Arsenic
      3. Solvents

  4. Organophosphorus Esters
  5. 2,4-Dichlorophenoxyacetic Acid
VI. References

KEY POINTS

- Clinical manifestations of neurologic dysfunction secondary to toxic exposure generally resemble those of primary neurologic disorders.
- Accurate differential diagnosis of neurologic disorder requires analysis of the work history.
- The mere exposure to a substance known to be capable of producing neurotoxic effects does not mean that each exposed individual will develop these reactions. Individual susceptibility as well as duration and intensity of exposure are the major factors involved in the development of a neurotoxic effect.
- Clinical manifestations of neurotoxic effects vary with the region of the nervous system affected. Central nervous system effects occur when a toxin reaches neuronal systems after passing the blood-brain barrier. Effects may be limited to the peripheral nervous system if the chemical molecules cannot pass this blood-brain barrier.
- Clinical manifestations of exposure are determined by the site of neurotoxicity.
- Disorders of peripheral nerves may be widespread and bilateral (polyneuropathy), and may include deficits in motor, sensory, sensorimotor, or autonomic function, and may be temporary or permanent. Electrodiagnostic studies are useful in the evaluation of peripheral nerve function.
- Central nervous system manifestations of neurotoxicity vary depending on different neurotoxicants and conditions of exposure, such as concentration of the toxicant, and duration and route of exposure. Symptoms may be due to acute or chronic exposure. Neuropsychiatric testing can aid in the diagnosis of central nervous system toxicity.
- Encephalopathy may result from exposure to lead, arsenic, manganese, mercury, organic solvents, and organophosphate insecticides. Parkinsonism may develop following exposure to certain neurotoxicants, including carbon monoxide, carbon disulfide, manganese, and N-methyl-4-phenyltetrahydropyridline (MPTP).
- Peripheral neuropathy may result from exposure to lead, arsenic, solvents, organophosphorus esters, and 2,4-dichlorophenoxyacetic acid (2,4-D). Numbness, tingling, weakness, and reduced reflexes are indicators of peripheral neuropathy.

QUESTIONS

1. Which is the most important factor that determines how neurotoxicity is expressed as clinical symptoms?

A. Anatomic site of the neurotoxic effect
B. Route of exposure
C. Nutritional state
D. Age at time of exposure
E. Previous injury

2. Which of the following may be attributed to trichloroethylene exposure?

A. Visual disturbances
B. Mental confusion
C. Fatigue and impaired concentration
D. Acute encephalopathy
E. All of the above

3. *Which of the following characteristics suggests small-fiber rather than large-fiber neuropathy?*

A. Loss of sensation to touch, pressure, and vibration
B. Loss of sensation to temperature and pain
C. Motor weakness
D. Loss of joint position sense
E. Absence of autonomic signs

4. *Which neuropsychological test(s) is (are) the most sensitive in individual cases of suspected occupational central neurotoxicity?*

A. Color vision
B. The Wechsler memory scale
C. Depression scale on the Minnesota Multiphasic Personality Inventory (MMPI)
D. Tests that cover many neurologic functions
E. Tests reflecting vigilance

5. *Which occupational toxic exposure is associated with a chronic movement disorder?*

A. Arsenic
B. Organophosphate toxicity
C. Organic solvents
D. Lead
E. Manganese

16

Noise-Induced Hearing Loss

OBJECTIVES

- Explain how noise can cause hearing loss
- State the normal range of human hearing
- Discuss audiometry
- List types of hearing protection devices
- Explain the components of a hearing conservation program

OUTLINE

I. Overview
   A. Noise in Industry
   B. Prevalence of Noise-Induced Hearing Loss
      Table 16–1. Summary of standard industrial classification (SIC) codes
   C. Roles and Challenges for Clinicians
   D. Example of Progressive Noise-Induced Hearing Impairment
      Table 16–2. Proportion of work force in industries in which noise levels
         may exceed 90 dB
      Table 16–3. Example of audiometric thresholds obtained on workers who
         exhibited progressive noise-induced hearing loss
II. Hearing and Noise
   A. Normal Hearing
   B. Nature of Damage to Hearing
   C. Differences Between Noise-Induced Temporary and Permanent Changes in
      Hearing
   D. Importance of Audiometric Changes Due to Noise
   E. Unilateral Versus Bilateral Loss
   F. Using Audiometric Monitoring Effectively
III. How to Identify Hazardous Noise Exposures
   A. Noise Measurements
   B. Behavioral Clues to Hazardous Noise
IV. Elements of an Occupational Hearing Conversation Program

    A. Education, Motivation, Supervision, and Discipline
    B. Assessment of Potentially Hazardous Exposures
    C. Assessing At-the-Ear Allowable Exposures for Those Wearing HPDs
    D. Monitoring Audiometry
    E. Personal Hearing Protection and Noise Control Measures
        Table 16–4. Types of audiometric examinations according to purpose of test
        Table 16–5. Classifications for basic types of personal protection devices
    F. Documentation of OHCP Monitorings
    G. Disposition and Follow-Up Actions
        Table 16–6. Considerations involved in choices of personal hearing protection devices
  V. Otologic/Audiologic Referral Criteria
  VI. Using Results of Audiometric Monitorings to Detect Noise-Induced Losses
    A. Comparing STS Between Current and Reference/Baseline Audiograms
    B. Comparing Threshold Shifts Between Sequential Audiograms
  VII. Accounting for Presbycusis (Aging)
        Table 16–7. Comparison of an annual and reference (baseline) where STS finding is negative
        Figure 16–1. Sample form for computing standard threshold shift (STS)
        Table 16–8. Results of sequential (longitudinal) audiometric monitoring revealing threshold shift trends before OSHA standard threshold shift achieved
  VIII. Correcting Noise-Induced Hearing Losses: Medical Alternatives
  IX. Nonauditory Effects of Noise
    A. Acute Acoustic Trauma
  X. References

KEY POINTS

- Cumulative overexposures to hazardous sounds and noises cause millions of people to lose hearing. Loss of hearing associated with overexposures are called noise-induced and such occurrences are mostly preventable.
- Since no treatment is available to mend noise-induced hearing loss, prevention measurements are paramount.
- Preplacement physical examinations should include audiometric examinations to discover noise-induced hearing loss prior to assigning a person to work in a noisy job.
- Audiometry, measuring hearing thresholds for different discrete pure-tone signals ranging from 500 to 6,000 or 8,000 hertz (Hz), furnishes valuable insight concerning the status of hearing. The lowest intensity level at which a sound (pure-tone signals) can be detected at a given test frequency is known as audiometric threshold, which is recorded in decibels (dB) with 0 to 25 dB considered in the normal range.
- The most critical frequency range for human audition is between 500 through 2,000 or 3,000 Hz—the range indispensable for hearing and understanding normal conversational speech.
- Millions of workers in the United States work in jobs in which noise exposures are 80 dB (A-weighted noise levels). Studies have demonstrated that approximately 33% of production workers have sustained some degree of hearing impairment.
- Excessive noise exposures damage the intricate microscopic structures within the inner ear, particularly those composing the organ of Corti.
- Observations of noise-induced hearing losses are classified into two categories: temporary and permanent. Noise-induced temporary threshold shifts (NITTS) are changes in hearing associated with transient overexposures to noise. Given an adequate period of auditory rest, hearing usually returns to preexposure levels. Noise-

induced permanent threshold shifts (NIPTS) refers to an irreversible condition in which, despite a prolonged period of auditory rest, hearing does not return to normal.

- Determining the effects of noise on hearing can be accomplished by serial audiometry.
- Although individual or area noise measurements may be used to evaluate the need for a hearing conservation program, there is a simple screening test to identify potentially hazardous noise. If a person needs to shout at a distance of about 1 m, the noise should be considered hazardous to unprotected ears.
- An occupational hearing conservation program should include (1) education, motivation, supervision, and discipline; (2) assessment of potentially hazardous noise exposures; (3) assessing at the ear allowable exposures for those wearing hearing protective devices (HPDs); (4) monitoring audiometry; (5) personal hearing protection and noise control measures; (6) documentation of monitoring; and (7) disposition and follow-up activities.
- Hearing protectors consist of three basic types: insert (devices that insert into the ear canal proper), semi-insert (devices covering the entry into the ear canal and held in place by a band or other type of suspension device), and muffs (devices completely encapsulating the auricle or pinna).
- Acute acoustic trauma may occur from unprotected exposure to very loud noise (about 140 dB), such as a ballistic blast or explosion. Clinical features may include vivid recall of the event, a sudden change in the status of hearing immediately following the encounter, possibly dizziness, and/or evidence of physical injury to the tympanic membrane.

QUESTIONS

1. Which frequency range is most important for comprehension of human speech?

A. >500
B. 500–3,000 Hz
C. 3,000–6,000 Hz
D. 6,000–8,000 Hz
E. all of the above

2. Which is the most effective and acceptable form of personal hearing protection?

A. Ear muffs
B. Foam ear plugs
C. Ear caps
D. Molded plastic ear plugs
E. The selection preferred by the worker from among the above

*3. Which of the following is **not** required as part of a hearing conservation program?*

A. Noise surveys
B. Personal hearing protection
C. Annual audiometric evaluations
D. Record-keeping system
E. Supervision by a physician

4. Which of the following may be a useful indicator to suggest that background noise is approaching the OSHA action levels of 85 dB?

A. Bilateral hearing losses
B. Temporary threshold shifts

C.   Necessity of shouting to be understood at 1-m distance
D.   Impaired comprehension of speech
E.   Audiometric abnormalities centered at 2,000 Hz

REFERENCES

Berger E, et al. (eds). *Noise and hearing conservation manual,* 4th ed. Akron, OH: American Industrial Hygiene Association, 1986.

Gasaway DC. *Hearing conservation: a practical manual and guide.* Englewood Cliffs, NJ: Prentice Hall, 1985.

Gasaway DC. Thirteen steps to developing an effective hearing protection program. *Plant Engineering* 41:51, February 26, 1987.

Royster JD, Royster LH. *Hearing conservation programs: practical guidelines for success.* Chelsea, MI: Lewis, 1990.

Suter AH, Franks JR, eds. *A practical guide to effective hearing conservation programs in the workplace.* Report no. 90-120. Cincinnati: U.S. Department of Health and Human Services, National Institute for Occupational Safety and Health, 1990.

17

Occupational Skin Disorders

OBJECTIVES

- Discuss skin conditions as the most common type of occupational illness
- List the two common types of occupational dermatitis
- State the uses and limitations of patch testing
- Explain the importance of exposure prevention and treatment of occupational skin disease

OUTLINE

    I. Significance of Occupational Dermatoses
   II. Evaluation of Occupational Dermatoses
         Table 17–1. Causes of occupational dermatoses
         Table 17–2. Common clinical expressions of occupational skin diseases
  III. History and Physical Examination
       A. Questions to Ask
       Table 17–3. Questions for a more effective history of occupational
          dermatoses
       B. Past Medical History
       C. Previous Contact Allergies
       D. Previous Jobs and Present Part-Time Jobs
       E. Hobbies
       F. Medications
       G. Physical Examination
  IV. Work-Site Evaluation
   V. The Role of Patch Testing
  VI. Exposure Prevention
       A. Engineering Controls
       B. Personal Protective Measures
       C. Administrative Controls
 VII. Treatment
       A. Topical Steroids

       B. Antihistamines
          Table 17–4. Topical steroids
       C. Prednisone
       D. Hand Dermatitis
  VIII. References
   IX. Appendix to Chapter 17: Some Occupations and Risk of Dermatitis

KEY POINTS

- Occupational dermatoses are those disorders of the skin caused by or made worse by the workplace environment. Skin disorders are one of the most common of all occupational illnesses and compose about 40% of all reported cases.
- Contact dermatitis is responsible for approximately 90% of these occupational skin afflictions.
- Irritant skin reactions are caused by substances that damage the skin at the site of contact by nonimmunologic mechanisms. Irritants are substances that cause injury to most individuals if given a sufficient concentration and time of exposure.
- Allergic contact reactions require a cell-mediated hypersensitivity mechanism, and generally a smaller number of workers are affected.
- Patch testing can be, in many instances, proof that sensitization has taken place that has resulted in allergic contact dermatitis. There is no scientific test to establish the presence of an irritant reaction.
- The first step in the evaluation of a potential occupational skin disease is to request that the worker bring in the material safety data sheets for all substances that may be used in his or her job duties.
- Allergic and irritant skin reactions generally cannot be differentiated by their clinical expression.
- A number of methods are available to help the worker avoid exposure to the offending agent if it has been determined that either an allergic contact dermatitis or an irritant contact reaction has occurred. These include engineering controls, personal protective measures, and administrative controls.
- All efforts should be made to keep the worker on the same job if measures appear to be available to prevent recurrences of the skin reaction.

QUESTIONS

*1. Regarding irritant dermatitis, which statement is **false?***

A. Patch tests are commonly used for diagnosis.
B. It is nonimmunologic in the mechanism of action.
C. Its clinical expression can look similar to allergic dermatitis.
D. Biopsies typically are not helpful in differentiating irritant from allergic dermatitis.
E. It is the most common expression of dermatitis in industry.

*2. Which statement is **false** regarding treatment of an occupational skin disorder?*

A. Topical high-potency corticosteroids should be used for eczematous eruptions.
B. Lubricants are used.
C. The more often a topical corticosteroid is used the more effective it is.
D. Long-term systemic prednisone is not appropriate to use to keep a worker on the job.
E. Systemic antihistamines are best used in conjunction with topical corticosteroids.

*3. Which statement is **false** regarding patch testing?*

A. Patch tests only reveal allergic reactions.

B. Patch tests are left on for 48 hours.
C. A final reading is typically made at 72–96 hours.
D. Only a limited number of test materials are available.
E. Chemicals in irritant concentration should be used when patch testing.

4. Clinical expressions of occupational skin diseases include:

A. eczematous dermatitis.
B. acneiform lesions.
C. pigmentary changes.
D. tumors.
E. all of the above.

5. Which statement is true about occupational skin eruptions?

A. most often occur on exposed skin
B. can occur first on covered areas of the body
C. often clear on weekends and vacations
D. over time can involve contiguous areas of skin
E. all of the above

18

Psychiatric Aspects of Occupational Medicine

OBJECTIVES

- Explain the relationships between occupation and mental status
- Discuss the effects of life events on mental status
- Explain mechanisms of posttraumatic stress disorder
- Explain the time shift syndrome and preventive strategies
- Classify the major groups of psychiatric disorders

OUTLINE

    I. Mental Status Examination
   II. Employee Assistance Programs
  III. Stress
          Table 18–1. The Holmes-Rahe Schedule of Recent Life Events
     A. Engaging the Patient as Your Ally
     B. Stress Management Techniques
        1. Time Management
        2. Relaxation Training
        3. Exercise
        4. Avocational Out Life Changes
        5. Spread Out Life Changes
        6. Group Stress Management Programs
   IV. Shift Work
     A. Acute Time Shift Syndrome
          Table 18–2. Guidelines on preventing the ill effect of shift work
     B. Chronic Shift Maladaptive Syndrome
    V. Malingering and Emotional Factors in Physical Symptoms (Somatoform Illness)
          Table 18–3. How to prevent jet lag
   VI. Posttraumatic Stress Disorder

VII. Common Psychiatric Disturbances that Affect Occupational Functioning
    A. Affective Disorders
    B. Psychotic Disorders
    C. Anxiety Disorders
    D. Personality Disorders
VIII. Mass Psychogenic Illness
  IX. Neuropsychiatric Disease Secondary to Toxic Exposure
    A. Multiple Chemical Sensitivities
   X. References

KEY POINTS

- An important tool of psychiatric diagnosis and evaluation is the mental status examination, an assessment of the patient's affect, appearance, speech pattern, thought processes, and cognition.
- Employee assistance programs (EAPs) encompass the coordinating efforts of a variety of counseling and psychological services designed to assist employees who have psychological or emotional problems that interfere with their work.
- Key aspects of EAPs include confidentiality, self-referral, and aggregate (not individual) reports.
- Stress refers not to a single event or reaction, but to a process that begins with a stressful event or series of events and ends with one's reaction to that event. Stressors can be divided into acute and chronic types.
- Research has shown a clear relationship between stress and productivity.
- An individual's relationship with stress may be influenced by his or her individual vulnerability, his or her life stage, and the particular stressor(s).
- Five commonly used techniques to manage stress are time management, relaxation training, physical exercise, avocational interests, and the spreading out of life changes.
- Shift work implies either long-term night work or work involving rotation between day, evening, and night shifts. Studies suggest that shift workers have increased morbidity and decreased work performance.
- The acute time shift syndrome (jet lag) commonly causes insomnia, gastrointestinal distress, sleepiness, and fatigue.
- The most commonly encountered consequence of shift work is a disturbance on the level of alertness.
- Somatoform disorders refer to the presence of symptoms that suggest physical disorders, but for which no organic basis can be established as the cause. Examples of somatoform disorders include conversion reactions, psychogenic pain, and hypochondriasis.
- The posttraumatic stress disorder (PTSD) is classified as an anxiety disorder. A subgroup of PTSDs has been described as atypical PTSDs, but closely resembles somatoform disorders.
- Neuropsychiatric symptoms may occur after human exposure to a variety of solvents, pesticides, and heavy metals. Individual vulnerability may vary. Acute intoxication may cause dizziness, light-headedness, and uncoordination. Chronic disorders may also occur and may produce mild to severe symptoms.
- Multiple chemical sensitivity is a condition in which the patient attributes multiple ill-defined symptoms (for which no organic cause can be found) to exposure to chemicals to which the patient claims to be allergic or hypersensitive. The symptoms may not be consistent with the accepted toxicologic properties of the offending agents. The intensity and range of symptoms are often in excess of those expected based on the patient's history. The etiology and pathology of this syndrome have yet to be determined.

QUESTIONS

1. Appropriate stress management techniques include:

A. exercise.
B. avocation.
C. time management.
D. relaxation techniques.
E. all of the above.

2. Acute time shift syndrome (jet lag) is assisted by the accommodation of

A. a phase delay of 2 hours.
B. a phase advance of 2 hours.
C. use of alcohol.
D. continuous low lighting.
E. none of the above.

3. Disturbance of a worker's circadian rhythm can result in:

A. disruption in sleep patterns.
B. gastrointestinal complaints.
C. decreased alertness.
D. increased incidence of cardiovascular disease.
E. all of the above.

4. A patient who is persistently delusional would most likely be diagnosed with

A. an anxiety disorder.
B. a psychotic disorder.
C. a neurosis.
D. a personality disorder.
E. malingering.

19

Allergy and Immunology

OBJECTIVES

- List the four types of hypersensitivity reactions
- Explain different manifestations of the onset of occupational asthma
- List the various types of occupational allergies
- Explain the workup of the hypersensitive patient
- Discuss the importance of avoidance of the offending agent in occupational allergy

OUTLINE

KEY POINTS

- Occupational allergic diseases include diseases of the skin, respiratory tract, and anaphylaxis. About 65,000 cases of occupational allergic respiratory disease are reported annually.

- Hypersensitivity reactions are based on the presence or absence of humoral antibodies, the types of antibodies involved, whether or not complement is required to drive the reaction to completion, the target organ, and the cell types involved.

- Type I (allergic or anaphylactic) reactions require immunoglobin E (IgE) antibody attached to mast cell receptors before antigen introduction. When an antigen cross-links with a specific antibody, the reaction causes release of histamine, serotonin, and other vasoactive amines from mast cell. These chemical mediators include the allergic reaction seen in allergic rhinitis, asthma, and anaphylaxis. A type I (allergic) reaction may occur immediately or it may be delayed for several hours (late-phase allergic reaction). Frequently a dual (immediate- and late-phase) reaction occurs. This delayed reaction can create confusion in evaluating the person with suspected occupational allergy.

- Type II reactions usually require immunoglobulin G (IgG) antibodies directed against antigen located on target cell surfaces. Complement may be needed to drive the antigen-antibody reaction, resulting in target cell destruction (immune hemolytic anemia, transfusion reaction, and some types of autoimmune disease).

- Type III (immune complex) reactions occur when excessive antigen causes a precipitation of antigen-antibody complex along vascular endothelium, resulting in subsequent attraction of polymorphonuclear leukocytes that cause local damage. Examples of this type of reaction include hypersensitivity pneumonitis and some autoimmune diseases.

- Type IV (delayed hypersensitivity) reactions require previously sensitized lymphocytes but no humoral antibodies nor complement. Antigens stimulate the lymphocytes to cause the release of lymphokines (interleukins and interferons). These lymphokines attract macrophages and leukocytes, which result in allergic contact dermatitis and granulomatous diseases such as tuberculosis.

- Laboratory studies are often inconclusive. The patient with asthma or eczema may have an elevated eosinophil count. The IgE level is not a good screening test for atopy. Skin testing remains the gold standard in determining the presence of specific IgE antibody. The radioallergosorbent test (RAST) or enzyme-linked immunosorbent assay (ELISA) may be alternatives to skin tests.

- Occupational rhinitis and rhinosinusitis may be irritative or allergic in nature. Irritation may occur following exposure to a variety of physical or chemical agents. Allergic reactions may result from exposures to high or low molecular weight antigens. Most high molecular weight antigens are naturally occurring, such as dust mites, fungal spores, animal danders, or foods. Low molecular weight agents, including a variety of organic chemicals (isocyanates, acid anhydrides, aldehydes) and inorganic chemicals (chromium, platinum), cause allergy through IgE-IgG human serum albumin hapten complexes or by poorly understood mechanisms.

- Occupational asthma is asthma caused by dusts, vapors, mists, and fumes in the workplace. Asthma caused by high molecular weight antigens is expressed either as an immediate or both an immediate and late reaction in over 95% of cases. Low molecular weight agents are associated with an isolated late reaction in about 50% of cases, greatly confounding the search for the causative agent.

- In the evaluation of suspected occupational asthma, it is suggested that (1) proof of airflow limitation is obtained; (2) hyperresponsiveness of the airways is detected; (3) the presence of atopy is evaluated; (4) the work-relatedness of asthma is suspected by a history of temporal association and pre- and postwork or serial expiratory flow or peak flow rates; and (5) consideration is given to the availability of skin tests or in vitro measurements of specific IgE antibodies.

- Hypersensitivity pneumonitis (extrinsic allergic alveolitis) occurs when inhaled allergens in the home or work environment causes a type III immunologic inflammatory reaction in the bronchioles, alveoli, and lung interstitium. The most frequent allergens are the thermophilic actinomycetes, which are found in warm, humid environments. Other causes may include the isocyanates and trimellitic anhydride.
- Acute bronchopulmonary aspergillosis is severe asthma associated with an elevated serum IgE and total eosinophil count. The condition results from colonization of the lower respiratory tract with fungi, usually *Aspergillus fumigatus* spores.
- Immediate and delayed hypersensitivity reactions to latex and natural rubber have been recently reported. True IgE mediated allergic reactions have caused severe anaphylactic reactions and deaths.
- Multiple chemical sensitivity (MCS) refers to a constellation of symptoms that involves multiple organ systems, resulting from exposure to extremely low doses of chemicals that customarily do not affect others. Symptoms may begin in a localized manner and then spread. Patients tend to have more disability than would be anticipated. There are no standard objective tests for this disorder. The diagnosis is based on history alone. The American Academy of Allergy and Immunology and the Council of Scientific Affairs of the American Medical Association have position statements to the effect that there are no well-controlled studies establishing a clear mechanism or cause for MCS. Both groups state that methods used by the clinical ecology proponents of MCS are unproven and experimental. A general approach to individuals with MCS is (1) to listen with an open mind, (2) do a complete initial exam, (3) do sufficient standard test to rule out any serious illness suggested by the history, (4) treat with reassurance and appropriate medications, (5) encourage physical and social interaction, and (6) refer to an appropriate specialist if needed.
- Immunotoxicology is the study of toxic effects of xenobiotics on the cellular and humoral components of the immune system. The majority of immunotoxicant chemicals are suppressive, either dampening the whole immune apparatus or acting at specific points. Regarding immunostimulation, various chemicals are capable of causing all types of hypersensitivity reactions.
- Because of the complexity of the numbers of chemicals and interactions, a logical system of testing is required. Such tier testing should be performed by certified immunologists at well-established, university-recognized immunotoxicologic laboratories.

QUESTIONS

*1. Hypersensitivity reactions can occur in all of the following **except:***

A. asthma.
B. tuberculosis.
C. beryllium disease.
D. multiple chemical sensitivity.
E. allergic contact dermatitis.

2. Fungal agents are capable of causing which of the following?

A. Hypersensitivity
B. Infection
C. Toxicity
D. All of the above
E. None of the above

3. *Chemical agents can have either a suppressive or stimulatory effect on the immune system. All of the following immunotoxicologic reactions have been associated with chemical exposure **except:***

A. asthma.
B. a scleroderma-like syndrome.
C. glomerulonephritis.
D. immune hemolytic anemia.
E. ankylosing spondylitis.

4. *Which of the following is true regarding latex hypersensitivity?*

A. Risk groups include rubber workers, health care workers, and patients with repeated surgeries or manipulations with catheters.
B. The route of exposure often determines the reaction type.
C. Reactions can vary from mild eczema to anaphylactic bronchospasms.
D. All of the above.
E. Only A and B above.

5. *Regarding multiple chemical sensitivity, which of the following is a **false** statement?*

A. Many patients identify a well-defined preceding event.
B. There are no consistent lab abnormalities.
C. A diagnosis is made after excluding other diseases.
D. An underlying mechanism has been established.
E. Usually no abnormal physical findings are present.

REFERENCES

Coombs RRA, Gell PGH, eds. *Clinical aspects of immunology.* Philadelphia: Lippincott, 1975:761.
Report of the Ad Hoc Committee on Environmental Hypersensitivity Disorders. Office of the Mister of Health, Toronto, Canada, 1989:17–18.

20

Arm Pain in the Workplace

OBJECTIVES

- List three common categories of musculoskeletal illness of the upper extremity.
- Discuss systemic diseases that may cause arm pain.
- Explain the differences and similarities between musculoskeletal disorders of the arm and cervical radiculopathies.
- Explain the frequency of soft tissue illness in the upper extremity.

OUTLINE

<ul style="list-style-type:none">
<li>I. Regional Musculoskeletal Illness That Can Be Ascribed to Osteoarthritis</li>
</ul>

    Table 20–1. Upper-extremity symptoms and/or signs that suggest a systemic cause

<ul style="list-style-type:none">
<li>II. The Neuropathic Syndromes</li>
</ul>

    Table 20–2. Signs and symptoms of cervical radiculopathies

    Table 20–3. Classic clinical features of an entrapment neuropathy

<ul style="list-style-type:none">
<li>III. Soft-Tissue Regional Musculoskeletal Illness at the Shoulder
  <ul style="list-style-type:none">
  <li>A. Soft-Tissue Illness</li>
  <li>B. Regional Musculoskeletal Illness of the Shoulder</li>
  <li>C. Regional Musculoskeletal Illness of the Elbow</li>
  <li>D. Regional Musculoskeletal Illness of the Wrist</li>
  <li>E. Regional Musculoskeletal Illness of the Hand</li>
  </ul>
</li>
<li>IV. When Is a Regional Musculoskeletal Illness of the Upper Extremity an Injury?</li>
<li>V. References</li>
</ul>

KEY POINTS

- Discomfort in the upper extremity is common. Regional musculoskeletal illness constitutes the vast majority of disorders of the upper extremity. There are three common categories of disorders in this region: illness that relates to osteoarthritis, illness as a consequence of neuropathy, and soft-tissue illness.

- Osteoarthritis of the proximal joints of the upper extremity (shoulder, elbow) is unusual. Osteoarthritis of the hands may cause the development of osteophytes (known as Heberden's nodes) of the distal interphalangeal joints. The proximal interphalangeal joints may also be involved (Bouchard's nodes). Arthritis of the first carpometacarpal joint is a common cause of pain at the base of the thumb. Forces are transduced during activities to the first carpometacarpal joint.
- Cervical radiculopathies are common and present with pain that, whether localized or radiating, is not usually exacerbated by limb motion. Unusual severity of pain, persistence beyond 6 weeks, suggestions of myelopathy (such as gait disorder, bowel or bladder dysfunction, Babinski's sign), or overt muscle weakness warrants additional diagnostic evaluation.
- Entrapment neuropathies have characteristic clinical features of the following:
  - Dysesthesias are localized to the sensory distribution of the nerve.
  - Discomfort and paresthesia are more prominent at rest than with usage.
  - Sensory fibers are more susceptible to insult than motor fibers (and therefore atropy is a late sign and an indication for surgical intervention).
  - Tinel's sign is frequently present.
  - Electrodiagnostic studies provide the gold standard for diagnosis.
- Soft-tissue illnesses represent the bulk of regional musculoskeletal disorders of the upper extremity. These patients have localized discomfort, tenderness, and often exacerbation with motion of the painful region. Their prognosis is excellent even though the symptoms can take months to remit. Tasks less likely to exacerbate symptoms can be proposed.

QUESTIONS

1. *A 55-year-old woman presents with a chief complaint of painful pinch located just distal to the radial styloid. Her examination is normal except for mild tenderness at that site. Which of the following is the likeliest diagnosis?*

A. Entrapment neuropathy involving the median nerve
B. Entrapment neuropathy involving the radial nerve
C. Osteoarthritis
D. deQuervain's tenosynovitis
E. Cervical radiculopathy

2. *Which of the following is normally associated with prolongation of sensory conduction in the median nerve at the wrist?*

A. Hyperthyroidism
B. Hypocalcemia
C. Obesity
D. Hypertension
E. deQuervain's tenosynovitis

3. *In cases of upper extremity entrapment neuropathy, which one of the following is* ***false?***

A. The most common is carpal tunnel syndrome.
B. Dysesthesias are localized to the sensory distribution of the nerve.
C. Dysesthesias often interrupt sleep.
D. Motor fibers are more susceptible to insult than sensory fiber.
E. Electrodiagnostic studies provide the gold standard.

4. *Which conditions usually involve nodule formation on tendons or fascia to the point of interference with finger function?*

A. Ganglion
B. Trigger finger
C. Dupuytren's contracture
D. Only B and C above
E. All of the above

REFERENCE

Nathan PA, et al. Obesity as a risk factor for slowing of sensory conduction of the median nerve in industry. *J. Occup. Med.* 34:379, 1992.

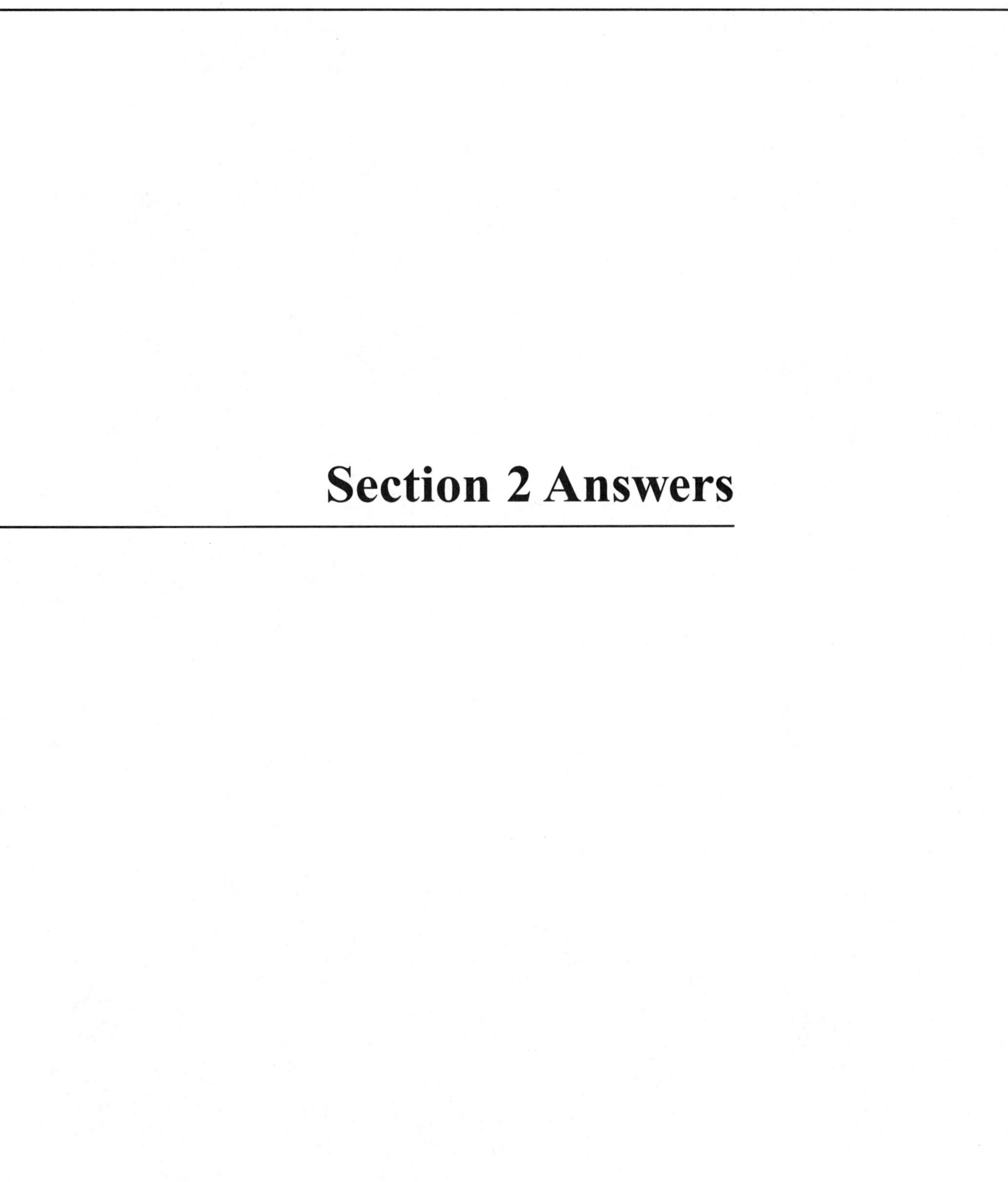

Section 2 Answers

CHAPTER 11 ANSWERS

1. The answer is E. (Reference: pp. 154–157)

The principal sites in the respiratory tract where different agents have the greatest effect are determined by their water solubility and particle size. Highly soluble agents dissolve readily in the secretions of the eyes, upper respiratory tract (nose, pharynx), and airways; less-soluble agents exert their main effects in the peripheral small airways and in the lung parenchyma. Particles greater than 10 μm tend to settle out in the upper-respiratory tract, those 3 to 10 μm settle mainly in the airways, and those less than 3 μm deposit mainly in the lung parenchyma and small airways.

Irritant agents that are relatively insoluble in water produce few upper respiratory or airway symptoms, and manifest themselves more insidiously.

The major symptom from these agents, however, is progressive breathlessness attributable to toxic pneumonitis with lung edema.

Long-term sequelae of toxic edema include lung fibrosis and occasionally bronchiolitis obliterans.

Another important sequela of acute exposures to lung irritants is a condition termed reactive airways dysfunction syndrome.

2. The answer is D. (Reference: pp. 160, 161)

Patients typically present with recurring episodes of fever, cough, headache, breathlessness, and general malaise that mimic acute infectious disease.

During the acute illness, the white cell count is elevated and generally shows a left shift; the sedimentation rate and serum immunoglobulins are also increased.

With repeated acute episodes, however, there may be progression to lung fibrosis with a restrictive ventilatory defect and a decreased diffusing capacity for carbon monoxide.

The pathogenesis of this group of disorders is traditionally thought to involve a type III (immune complex) response to inhaled antigens.

The outlook for most patients with one of these forms of extrinsic allergic alveolitis is good if they present before lung fibrosis is extensive and if they cease being exposed to the offending agent(s). Corticosteroid therapy may help accelerate recovery.

3. The answer is B. (Reference: p. 148)

Respiratory impairment is assigned primarily in terms of abnormal spirometry. By convention, ventilatory abnormalities are described either as being obstructive (defined as an abnormally decreased FEV_1 and decreased FEV_1/FVC ratio) or restrictive (an abnormally decreased FVC, with well-preserved FEV_1/FVC ratio).

4. The answer is C. (Reference: pp. 151–154)

Lung function is typically well preserved in workers with simple silicosis. Once conglomeration occurs, however, lung function is frequently impaired, and functional deterioration may be rapid.

Chronic cough and phlegm (chronic bronchitis) are common symptoms among workers with heavy silica exposure and those who have silicosis. Phlegm production generally increases in advanced stages of silicosis; recurrent bacterial infections are common.

It is now apparent that coal alone in combination with smoking can cause emphysema in workers with moderate to severe coal worker's pneumoconiosis (CWP). Coal workers frequently have a cough and phlegm, which are often accompanied by mild reductions in forced expiratory flows.

Diagnosis of asbestosis is not as simple as that for silicosis or CWP. Unlike the other two disorders, mild or early asbestosis is relatively more difficult to detect with a chest x-ray. The first changes are usually irregular linear densities that are seen initially at the lung bases but increase in number, coarseness, and extent as the disease progresses. Lung function changes may precede the radiographic changes, with the most prominent early effects being a decrease in FVC and a decrease in the diffusing capacity for carbon monoxide. When other findings are normal, an important clue to possible interstitial disease is the presence of inspiratory rales at the lung bases.

Tin, barium, antimony, and titanium cause radiodense nodules that are collections of dust-filled macrophages with no fibrotic reaction. These dusts are among a group of agents that have been termed inert dusts because they deposit in the lungs but elicit little fibrosis reaction.

5. The answer is E. (Reference: pp. 157–159)

Nonimmune mechanisms are important, particularly for highly reactive chemicals of low molecular weight.

Although many patients experience typical recurrent episodes of wheezing and breathlessness, in some the onset of symptoms may develop more insidiously and may not show typical acute episodic attacks.

Symptoms may not be obviously work related: a sizable fraction of workers with occupational asthma experience their symptoms mainly in the evenings or at night. Also, following exposures to some occupational causes of asthma (e.g., western red cedar, toluene diisocyanate), the recovery period may take several days or weeks.

Asthma may be precipitated in some cases by minute levels of the responsible agent(s).

CHAPTER 12 ANSWERS

1. The answer is E. (Reference: p. 166)

Significant risk factors for disabling back injury include previous back injury claims; job dissatisfaction; poor ratings from supervisors; repetitive, boring tasks; younger age and shorter duration of employment; smoking; and a history of non–back injury claims.

2. The answer is D. (Reference: p. 167).

Major risk factors for prolapsed disk include frequent lifting of objects heavier than 25 lb, exposure to whole body vibration, cigarette smoking, and narrow lumbar vertebral canals.

3. The answer is B. (Reference: p. 168)

Plain films of the lumbosacral spine are of limited value in the diagnosis of acute back pain, unless there is clinical suspicion of vertebral fracture, primary or metastatic cancer, or infection (osteomyelitis).

4. The answer is D. (Reference: pp. 169, 170)

The cornerstones of treatment for low back pain arising from a work-related episode are rest and symptomatic relief of the discomfort. Although the precise amount of bed rest that is necessary to promote relief of low back pain is debatable, a recent study suggests no difference in outcome (period of recovery) between the recommendation of 2 or 7 days of bed rest.

Within the first 24 hours of acute pain, ice applied to the area of discomfort can be helpful.

In many cases of acute back pain, muscle spasm occurs, for which administration of a muscle relaxant can afford relief. The use of nonsteroidal antiinflammatory agents can also aid in symptomatic relief.

CHAPTER 13 ANSWERS

1. The answer is B. (Reference: p. 188)

Some carcinogens, such as bis(chloromethyl)ether, can damage DNA directly, but most require metabolic activation by enzymes.

The enzymes primarily responsible for this activation are those of the cytochrome P-450 system (Gonzalez et al., 1991). Others include *N*-acetyltransferase, epoxide hydolase, and glutathione S-transferase. The primary function of these enzymes is to render xenobiotics more polar and therefore more readily excretable. However, their products are often reactive electrophiles, which can bond with DNA to cause adducts, and result in mutations.

2. The answer is C. (Reference: pp. 188, 189)

Several arguments in support of thresholds have been advanced. First, there are known repair mechanisms that correct DNA damage, at least at low levels of exposure. Second, certain carcinogens, such as trace elements and hormones, are ubiquitous and even essential at low doses; it is argued that these substances are carcinogenic only at higher doses. Third, factors that act epigenetically, such as promoters that stimulate cell divisions, often have reversible effects, implying a threshold phenomenon.

Finally, certain empiric data have been interpreted to be consistent with the existence of thresholds.

3. The answer is A. (Reference: p. 189)

Epidemiologic studies are potentially the most definitive source of information on human carcinogenicity, since they are based on human exposures in "real-life" situations.

4. The answer is A. (Reference: p. 191)

The IARC has evaluated approximately 750 chemicals, industrial processes, and personal habits. More than 50 have been placed in group 1.

5. The answer is B. (Reference: pp. 194, 195)

Cancer surveillance in occupational settings has been best explored with regard to bladder and lung cancers.

For bladder cancer two methods have been primarily used—urinalysis for microscopic hematuria and urine cytology, which is relatively sensitive in detecting both superficial and invasive bladder cancer.

NIOSH, in 1989, concluded that urinalysis and cytology might be appropriate, especially following high exposure to known or suspected bladder carcinogens.

Lung cancer surveillance consists of interval chest radiography or sputum cytology, or both.

Results, in combination with other data, have supported the recommendations that no routine surveillance for lung cancer be offered, even to the high-risk populations. Other kinds of medical surveillance for occupational cancer are also not recommended.

CHAPTER 14 ANSWERS

1. The answer is E. (Reference p. 204)

In general, over 80% of people who suffer an MI or undergo CABG surgery return to their original positions. The major adverse medical prognosticators for failure to return to work include left ventricular dysfunction and persistence of ischemia.

In a review of 893 men who underwent a CABG, the major factor involved in return to work was the type of job. Age plays an important role.

Those who worked prior to surgery tended to work thereafter.

Relief of anginal pain is another factor.

One's level of self-assessed disability may affect ability to return to work.

Psychological factors play a very important role in return to work after a cardiac event.

2. The answer is B. (Reference p. 208)

The American College of Cardiology has suggested that telemetry be employed when the following conditions exist: (1) severely depressed left ventricular function (ejection fraction < 30%); (2) resting complex ventricular arrhythmia (Lown type 4 or 5); (3) ventricular arrhythmias appearing or increasing with exercise; (4) previous cardiac arrest; (5) after MI complicated by congestive heart failure, cardiogenic shock, or serious ventricular arrhythmias; (6) severe CAD and marked exercise-induced ischemia (ST segment depression >2 mm); or (7) inability to self-monitor heart rate due to physical or intellectual impairment (American College of Cardiology, 1986).

3. The answer is E. (Reference pp. 209, 210)

Carbon monoxide can cause headaches, light-headedness, and dizziness as well as chest pain secondary to myocardial ischemia.

The major cardiovascular risk of solvents appears to be dysrhythmias.

Carbon disulfide, a substance used in the viscose rayon industry, has been associated with increasing the rate of atherosclerosis.

Table 14–3. *Guidelines for patient referral based on cholesterol levels*

Classification	Cholesterol level	LDL cholesterol level
High	≥240 mg/100 ml	≥160 mg/100 ml
Borderline high	200–239 mg/100 ml	130–159 mg/100 ml
Desirable	<200 mg/100 ml	<130 mg/100 ml

The National Cholesterol Education Program (NCEP) panel developed the following guidelines for referral based on blood cholesterol level:

Classification	Recommended action
High (≥240 mg/100 ml)	Refer to physician for follow-up[a]
Borderline high	Refer to physician for follow-up [a] if history of coronary heart disease or if two or more other CHD risk factors (excluding high-density lipoprotein cholesterol) detected on interview; if no reported history of CHD or less than two risk factors, refer to physician within 1 year for repeat cholesterol measurement
Desirable (<200 mg/100 ml)	Recommended a repeat cholesterol follow-up in 5 years

[a]Individuals should be seen by their physician with 2 months.
CHD, congestive heart disease; LDL, low-density lipoprotein.
Source From NCEP *Report on population strategies for blood cholesterol reduction.* Washington, DC US Department of Health and Human Services, 1990, pp 8, 30.

Occupational exposure to nitrogylcerin and other aliphatic nitrates has been associated with angina-like pain, MI, and cardiovascular death.

This manifestation is presumed to be due to rebound coronary spasm as a result of withdrawal of nitrates.

4. The answer is E. (Reference: p. 201, Table 14–3)

Despite potential inaccuracies in measurement of serum cholesterol levels, the National Cholesterol Education Program (NCEP) recommends the classification shown in Table 14–3, based on total and LDL cholesterol levels (NCEP, 1990).

CHAPTER 15 ANSWERS

1. The answer is A. (Reference: p. 215)

Clinical manifestations of neurotoxic effects depend on the region of the nervous system that is affected.

Clinical manifestations are determined by the site of neurotoxicity.

2. The answer is E. (Reference: p. 215)

Disorders of peripheral nerves are manifested clinically by a decrease in the ability to perceive sensation, spontaneous sensations (tingling), and painful sensations (dysesthesiae).

3. The answer is B. (Reference: p. 216)

In small fiber neuropathy there is relative preservation of motor power and sensory functions of touch-pressure, vibration, and joint sensation.

Sensations of pain and temperature are usually lost in small-fiber neuropathy. In large-fiber neuropathy, there is weakness as well as loss of sensation of position, vibration, and touch-pressure.

4. The answer is D. (Reference: p. 217)

In clinical situations, it is generally more appropriate to select neuropsychological tests that will assess as many functions as possible. These tests include attention (including vigilance, as well as ability to hold and manipulate information), motor skills and reaction time, concept formation (reasoning), language, visuospatial abilities, and mood and personality.

5. The answer is E. (Reference: p. 221)

Neurotoxicity of manganese was recognized after manganese miners developed irritability, nervousness, and emotional lability. Some experienced visual and auditory hallucinations, whereas others had compulsive, repetitive, and uncontrollable actions.

The final established phase exhibits muscular rigidity, fine tremors, and a cock walk.

CHAPTER 16 ANSWERS

1. The answer is B. (Reference: p. 230)

The most critical frequency range for human audition is between 500 through 2,000 or 3,000 Hz—the range indispensable for hearing and understanding normal conversational speech.

2. The answer is E. (Reference: pp. 238, 239)

No single type is best for all users, and many factors affect overall functional compatibility and effectiveness (Berger et al., 1986; Gasaway, 1985, 1987).

OSHA and others recommend that employees be allowed to make selections from two or more types of appropriate devices.

3. The answer is E. (Reference: p. 236)

An occupational hearing conservation program should contain specific and well-defined functional elements: (1) education, motivation, supervision, and discipline; (2) assessment of potentially hazardous noise exposures; (3) assessing at-the-ear allowable exposures for those wearing HPDs; (4) monitoring audiometry; (5) personal hearing and protection and noise control measures; (6) documentation of OHCP monitorings; and (7) disposition and follow-up actions (Gasaway, 1985; Royster and Royster, 1990; Suter and Franks, 1990).

4. The answer is C. (Reference: p. 236)

A simple technique for identifying a potentially unprotected hazardous noise is based on observation. If a person needs to shout at a distance of about 1 m (about 3 feet), the noise should be considered hazardous to unprotected ears, an indicator of when either on-or-off-the-job auditory risks are encountered that equal or exceed about 85 dB (Gasaway, 1985).

CHAPTER 17 ANSWERS

1. The answer is A. (Reference: pp. 249, 250)

Irritant contact dermatitis represents 80% of all the contact dermatitis problems of industry. Irritant reactions are caused by substances that damage the skin at the site of contact by nonimmunologic mechanisms. Irritants, in general, are substances that cause injury to most individuals if given sufficient concentration and time of exposure.

Patch testing can be, in many instances, proof that sensitization has taken place that has resulted in allergic contact dermatitis.

Allergic and irritant skin reactions generally cannot be differentiated by their clinical expressions. Both may have similar skin changes. Skin biopsies are also not generally useful.

2. The answer is C. (References: pp. 256. 257)

Occupational physicians are advised to become familiar with the broad range of topical steroid creams and to use high-potency steroids when appropriate.

In addition to topical steroids, the skin needs lubrication between applications of the steroid cream.

Topical steroids may become less effective if applied more than three times per day.

To avoid sedation of the worker from the use of antihistamines, it is advisable to use potent topical steroids that have their own antipruritic effect.

As with high-potency topical steroid, systemic prednisone therapy should not be given as a means of keeping a worker on the job when the environment in the cause of the persistent skin problems.

3. The answer is E. (Reference: p. 255)

Patch tests reveal only allergic contact sensitization and cannot be used to determine the presence of an irritant contact dermatitis. Patch testing involves a standardized application of chemicals (in a nonirritating concentration) onto the skin of the patient. Either strips of cellulose disks (Al-test) or aluminum chambers (Finn Chambers) are applied to the skin, generally to the back for 48 hours, after which the test strips are removed and the areas examined. The test sites are reevaluated again after an additional 48 hours.

4. The answer is E. (Reference: Table 17–2, pp. 253, 254)

Other skin disorders such as psoriasis should always be considered in the differential diagnosis.

Idiopathic lichen planus can also be confused with occupational skin eruptions.

A complete skin examination is necessary to determine the presence of other dermatologic conditions, such as psoriasis, lichen planus, or eczema.

5. The answer is E. (Reference: pp. 251, 252)

Many occupational skin eruptions begin on exposed skin. However, as a dermatitis persists, it may involve contiguous areas of skin and distant sites, a process known as autoeczematization or an id reaction.

Not all occupational skin disorders develop in exposed sites.

In many cases of an occupational contact dermatitis, the eruption worsens as the workweek progresses and stabilizes or lessens on weekends and vacations.

CHAPTER 18 ANSWERS

1. The answer is E. (Reference: pp. 270, 271)

Stress management techniques:

Time management
Relaxation training
Exercise
Avocational interests
Spread-out life changes

2. The answer is A. (Reference: p. 271)

Our circadian system can adapt to a phase delay of 2 hours or a phase advance of a half-hour without much disruption.

3. The answer is E. (Reference: p. 272)

Disturbance of the worker's biologic clock or circadian rhythms is responsible for a shift maladaptation syndrome.

The most common effects include gastrointestinal and cardiovascular disturbances and effects on level of alertness.

Night shift or rotating shift workers are more likely to suffer from insomnia and difficulty staying awake at work.

4. The answer is B. (Reference: p. 275)

Psychosis implies a severe psychiatric disturbance in which the patient is out of touch with reality, which leads to an inability to function in daily life. The most common psychotic disorder is schizophrenia.

CHAPTER 19 ANSWERS

1. The answer is D. (Reference: p. 279)

Proposed in 1995, the Gell and Coombs classification of hypersensitivity reactions (Coombs and Gell, 1975) still remains the standard guide for types of immune responses. The four types of reactions are based on the presence of absence of humoral antibodies, the type of antibodies involved, whether or not complement is required to drive the reaction to completion, the target organ, and the cell types involved.

Type I: the allergic reaction seen in allergic rhinitis, asthma, and anaphylaxis.

Type II: results in target cell destruction (immune hemolytic anemia, transfusion reaction, and some types of autoimmune disease).

Type III: examples of this type of reaction are hypersensitivity pneumonitis and some autoimmune diseases.

Type IV: results in allergic contact dermatitis.

2. The answer is D. (Reference: p. 286)

Of all the microbiologic agents, the fungi present particular problems, not only because of their ubiquity (greatest source of aeroallergens worldwide), but also because of their ability to cause hypersensitivity, infection, and toxicity.

3. The answer is E. (Reference: p. 290)

Although the majority of immunotoxicants have a suppressive effect, some may stimulate the immune mechanism.

Some metals (nickel, platinum, and beryllium) are capable of causing asthma.

Isocyanates can cause asthma. Dieldrin pesticide is associated with immune hemolytic anemia , hydrazine with lupus-like syndrome, monomeric vinyl chloride with scleroderma-like changes, and heavy metals (such as gold) with immune complex glomerulonephritis.

Benzine, specifically causes the reduced synthesis of IgG and IgE antibodies.

4. The answer is D. (Reference: p. 285)

Several groups are at greatest risk: (1) health care workers and workers in the rubber industry, (2) children with meningomyelocele or urogenital abnormalities who have undergone numerous manipulations with catheters and surgeries, and (3) any individuals who have a history of past latex reactions, a history of hand dermatitis from contact with latex, and a general atopic history, and those who have had unexplained anaphylactic reactions during surgery.

5. The answer is D. (Reference: pp. 287, 288)

Upon physical exam, the patient is usually free from any abnormal or objective findings (Office of the Minister of Health, 1989).

The symptom complex is usually identified by a well-defined event—exposure to pesticides, petrochemicals, or generally innocuous substances.

Because there are no standard objective tests that show a consistent abnormality in MCS, the diagnosis is based on history alone.

There are no well-controlled studies establishing a clear mechanism or cause for the multiple chemical sensitivity syndrome.

CHAPTER 20 ANSWERS

1. The answer is C. (Reference: p. 294)

Osteoarthritis of the hands, however, is common. The process afflicts all of us as we age but is most frequent and more advanced in the postmenopausal woman.

The principal occupationally related compromise to which these women are at risk relates to power pinch.

Osteoarthritis of the first carpometacarpal joint is a far more common cause of discomfort at the base of the thumb tunnel syndrome or tendonitis in women beyond middle age.

2. The answer is C. (Reference: p. 295)

Conduction in the median nerve is normally delayed as a function of aging and obesity, particularly in women (Nathan et al., 1992).

3. The answer is D. (Reference: Table 20–3, p. 294)

Entrapment neuropathies of the upper extremities are far less frequent than cervical radiculopathies. Most are rare indeed. The most common is carpal tunnel syndrome.

4. The answer is D. (Reference: p. 297)

Dupuytren's contractures are as common as trigger fingers and result in hyperplasia and hypertrophy of the palmar fascia with fibrotic nodule formation.

Section 3

21

Suspecting Occupational Disease

OBJECTIVES

- Explain the importance of work-related etiologies in the differential diagnosis
- Discuss the extent of occupational illness in the United States
- Explain obstacles to physicians in the recognition of work-related health problems
- List contributions that physicians have made in the identification of previously unrecognized occupational diseases
- Illustrate an organized four-step approach to history-taking and diagnosis of occupational or environmental illness
- Identify examples of environmental causes of medical problems
- Identify examples of common dangerous household products
- Identify examples of hazards in hobbies
- List occupational sentinel health events

OUTLINE

KEY POINTS

- Patients suffering from work-related illness enter physicians' offices daily, but diseases of occupational etiology are rarely included in the differential diagnosis. It is difficult to estimate the extent of work-related disease in the United States because of the lack of accurate information, but in 1990 such cases increased to nearly 6.8 million cases identified by the Bureau of Labor Statistics (BLS). These figures do not include small companies, farmers, or government workers. The majority of work-related illnesses are associated with repetitive motion.
- It is believed that the lack of recognition of work-related health problems by practitioners may be due to insufficient education. In a 1983 survey, only 50% of medical schools taught courses in occupational medicine, and the average curriculum time was 4 hours.
- The clinical manifestations of occupational disease may be identical to the signs and symptoms of other disease. Some work-related diseases have a latency period of many years.
- Physicians can enhance their ability to recognize work-related disease by taking a good occupational history. They should routinely ask for a short list of current and past longest held jobs with a brief description of potential hazards. A key question in the review of symptoms is, Are you now (or have you ever been) exposed to fumes, chemicals, dust, loud noise, or radiation? One should ask about any temporal relationship between activities in the home or job and the chief complaint.
- A sentinel health effect (SHE) is a disease, disability, or untimely death that is occupationally related and whose occurrence may provide the impetus for epidemiologic industrial hygiene surveys or serve as a warning signal that material substitution, engineering control, personal protection, or medical care may be required.
- Exposure to the occupational environment may aggravate underlying medical conditions. For example, carbon monoxide may precipitate anginal symptoms in patients with coronary artery disease.
- Sources of toxic contamination may include neighborhood pollution from chronic low-level contamination, household chemicals, hobbies, and industrial effluents emitted into the air or water.
- To characterize a chemical exposure, it is necessary to identify the chemicals that might have caused symptoms, or a description of the dust involved. In the case of radiation, it is necessary to determine the form. In addition, one must ask about handling and protective measures used by the patient. Finally, one must consider the mode of entry (ingestion, inhalation, etc.).
- It is helpful to obtain a Material Safety Data Sheet from the worker or the employer in order to determine the generic ingredients.

QUESTIONS

1. Which one of the following is correct?

A. In 1990, according to the BLS, the number of occupational injuries and illnesses decreased for the first time.
B. In the 1990 BLS report, the majority of new cases of occupational illnesses were related to repetitive motions, such as vibrations and repeated pressures.
C. The BLS data probably overestimate the number of occupational injuries and illnesses.
D. The number of cancer deaths caused by occupational exposure is precisely known.
E. The BLS reports statistics for all U.S. employers.

2. Which of the following contribute to the underrecognition of work-related health problems by physicians?

A. Insufficient education

B. Lack of uniqueness
C. Long latency periods
D. All of the above
E. None of the above

3. *Dr. Goldman describes a four-step approach for a physician to use for history taking and diagnosis of occupational or environmental illness. Which one of the following is **not** correct?*

A. Step 1, the Occupational History Survey, need only be done for patients with complaints suggestive of an occupational or environmental etiology.
B. Step 2, Defining Sources of Exposure, should be done for any patient with an affirmative response from step 1.
C. Step 2 includes defining sources of exposure at home as well as at work.
D. Step 3, Identification and Description of Hazard, includes determining the chemical and physical forms of agents, describing how these agents or substances are handled, and determining potential modes of entry.
E. Step 4, Follow-up, Consultation, and Resolution of the Problem, may be the development of a final opinion or a request for additional help.

4. *Which one of the following is correct with regard to the Occupational History Survey (Step 1)?*

A. You need only list the patient's current job.
B. Never ask, "Are you now (or have you ever been) exposed to fumes, chemicals, dust, loud noise, or radiation?"
C. It is important to inquire about temporal relationships between the onset of symptoms and the performance of tasks at work and at home.
D. A temporal relationship between symptoms and nonwork activities excludes a relationship with work.
E. The Occupational History Survey is the basis for your final opinion on any exposure-disease relationship.

5. *Step 2, Defining Sources of Exposure, differs from step 1 because the physician*

A. Lists all jobs, not just the current and longest held jobs, for the patient.
B. Obtains brief descriptions of the operations performed by the patient on the job.
C. Inquires about methods of chemical absorption.
D. Reviews standards of personal protective equipment.
E. Does not inquire about illnesses in other workers.

REFERENCES

Bureau of Labor Statistics. *Results of Bureau of Labor Statistics survey on U.S. occupational injuries, illnesses in 1990.* Washington, DC: US Department of Labor, 1991.

Levy BS. The teaching of occupational health in United States medical schools: 5 year follow-up of an initial survey. *Am. J. Public Health* 75:79, 1985.

Rossol M. *The artist's complete health and safety guide.* New York: Allworth Press, 1990.

22

Industrial Hygiene

OBJECTIVES

- Identify ways that an industrial hygienist may help a physician considering health risks associated with work settings
- State the goals of industrial hygiene
- Distinguish the types of hazards found in the workplace
- List types, methods, and expression of results of monitoring
- Explain sources of exposure guidelines
- Identify sources of industrial hygiene services

OUTLINE

    I. Types of Hazards
       A. Gases and Vapors
       B. Dusts
       C. Fumes and Mists
       D. Physical Agents
       E. Biologic Agents
   II. Monitoring
           Figure 22–1. A passive dosimeter badge
           Figure 22–2. Air sampling equipment
       A. Gases and vapors
           Figure 22–3. A colorimetric detector
           Figure 22–4. Direct-reading instrument
       B. Dusts
       C. Fumes and Mists
       D. Physical Agents
       E. Biologic Agents
 III. Exposure Guidelines
           Table 22–1. Recognized exposure guidelines
           Table 22–2. Airborne chemicals for which biologic exposure indices (BEI) have been adopted

Table 22–3. Airborne chemicals for which biologic exposure indices (BEI)
have been proposed
IV. Industrial Hygiene Services
V. References

KEY POINTS

- The profession of industrial hygiene has as its main goal the recognition, evaluation, and control of workplace health hazards. Recognition of a hazard requires knowledge of both the processes and the materials used in the processes.
- The hazards found in the workplace can be divided into five types: gases/vapors, dusts, fumes/mists, physical agents, and biologic agents.
- Gases are substances that are normally in the gaseous state at room temperature; in contrast, vapors are the gaseous state of substances that are normally in the liquid state at room temperature. The main route of entry into the body for both gases and vapors is through inhalation.
- A variety of dust types may be found in the workplace, including nuisance-type dusts, toxic dusts, and pneumoconiosis-producing dusts.
- A fume is a solid that has been vaporized and subsequently condenses. In welding steel, for example, iron oxide fume is produced. A mist is a liquid that has been dispersed into the air as fine droplets.
- Physical agents encountered in the workplace may include noise, heat, cold, ionizing and nonionizing radiation, and vibration.
- More recently, biologic agents, including bacteria, viruses, and fungi, are being evaluated by industrial hygienists.
- The industrial hygienist monitors employee exposure to air contaminants. This can be done by obtaining personal or area samples. Personal samples are obtained by placing the sampling device and/or equipment on the worker. In area sampling, apparatus is placed in the vicinity of the worker performing the job.
- Organic gases and vapors can be collected with an absorbing material, such as silica gel or activated charcoal. The concentration is determined based on the time the device was exposed to air and the amount of contaminant. Dusts may be monitored by a variety of instruments. The most common method is to collect the dust on a filter medium using an air sampling pump. Fumes and mists are collected on filters, like dusts, and analyzed in a laboratory. Physical agents such as noise and microwaves are measured with electronic instruments which respond to the energy field of the agent.
- There are several guidelines that are used by the industrial hygienist to evaluate the significance of exposure levels to air contaminants. The American Conference of Governmental Industrial Hygienists (ACGIH) publishes threshold limit values (TLVs) annually. These are meant to protect nearly all workers from adverse effects when they are repeatedly exposed to an agent 8 hours a day, 5 days a week for a working lifetime. If a worker's exposure to an agent is below the guidelines, one cannot necessarily conclude that the exposure is safe for that person or that his or her symptoms are not necessarily related to the exposure.
- The Biologic Exposure Indices (BEIs), also published by ACGIH, are warning levels of biologic response to a chemical or its metabolite. They are concentrations of a chemical or its metabolite usually in either blood or urine that appear to reflect levels that are safe to human health.
- The OSHA permissible exposure limits (PELs) are published in the Code of Federal Regulations.
- Although most exposure limits are defined as 8-hour time-weighted averages, other values refer to ceiling limits. Ceiling values, which should never be exceeded, are usually assigned to strong irritants, cardiac sensitizers, and carcinogens. Another limit value is the short-term exposure limit (STEL).

- If a patient has symptoms or an illness that is suspected to be due to the workplace, industrial hygiene data should be reviewed, if available. Such data may be available from many sources. OSHA offices, workers' compensation insurance carriers, or others may have conducted investigations of facilities and have monitoring data.

QUESTIONS

*1. Which one of the following is **not** a goal of industrial hygiene?*

A. Recognition of potential hazards in the workplace
B. Evaluation of potential hazards in the workplace
C. Evaluation of workers exposed to potential hazards in the workplace
D. Control of potential hazards in the workplace
E. Anticipation of potential hazards in the workplace

2. Burning is a common task in the fabrication of metal products. In burning, a hot flame from an oxygen-acetylene (oxyacetylene) torch is used to cut metal. Which one of the following is correct?

A. Acetylene and oxygen are vapors.
B. Metal oxides are gases.
C. Metal oxides are mists.
D. Metal oxides are fumes.
E. Metal oxides are dusts.

*3. Which of the following is **incorrect?***

A. The American Conference of Governmental Industrial Hygienists (ACGIH) publishes threshold limit values (TLVs).
B. The Occupational Safety and Health Administration publishes permissible exposure limits (PELs).
C. The National Institute for Occupational Safety and Health (NIOSH) publishes recommended exposure limits (RELs).
D. The American Industrial Hygiene Association (AIHA) publishes Biologic Exposure Indices (BEIs).
E. Even though the individual airborne concentrations of a mixture of chemicals do not exceed recommended guidelines (TLVs or PELs), it is possible that the equivalent exposure for the mixture may suggest overexposure.

4. What is a permissible exposure limit (PEL)?

A. An air contaminant concentration level used by the EPA
B. An air contaminant concentration level that is the same as a TLV
C. An air contaminant concentration level used by OSHA that is the upper limit of employee exposure acceptability
D. An air contaminant concentration level used to determine the acceptability of chemical emissions to the atmosphere
E. An air contaminant concentration level that is considered safe to exceed

5. How are industrial hygienists involved in occupational health?

A. They manage workers' compensation claims.
B. They are like physician's assistants.
C. They recognize, evaluate, and control sanitation problems in the workplace.
D. They recognize, evaluate, and control health hazards in the workplace.

E. They do stack testing for industrial emissions to determine compliance with EPA regulations.

6. *An industrial hygienist informs you that an overexposure to lead is occurring in the machining area. Which one of the following control strategies should be taken immediately?*

A. Open all windows and doors to dilute the lead dust in the air.
B. Shut down the operation until a long-term control strategy can be devised.
C. Tell the company to stop using lead.
D. Hire another industrial hygienist for a second opinion.
E. Shut down the operation until the employees are provided with the appropriate respiratory protection.

7. *What is the Biologic Exposure Index (BEI)?*

A. A warning level of biologic response to a chemical or metabolite
B. The OSHA exposure limit for employee exposure to air contaminants in the workplace
C. The same as a threshold limit value
D. An exposure index used to evaluate a work group's biologic response to a chemical
E. An exposure index used by industrial hygienists to evaluate an employee's exposure to microbiologic contaminants in the workplace air

23

Toxicology

OBJECTIVES

- State general toxicologic principles and definitions
- List the factors that characterize exposure
- Explain factors that affect the absorption of toxicants
- List factors that affect the distribution of toxicants
- Identify the two major types of chemical transformations and factors that affect them
- Explain factors that affect the excretion of toxicants
- Identify standard animal toxicity testing methods
- State the potential application of animal toxicity tests to clinical situations
- Discuss the use of the MSDS to obtain toxicologic information

OUTLINE

I. Exposure Considerations
   A. Routes of Contact
   B. Dose
   C. Duration and Frequency of Exposure
II. Absorption, Distribution, Metabolism, and Excretion
   A. Absorption Through the Lung
   B. Absorption Through the Skin
   C. Absorption Through the Gastrointestinal Tract
   D. Absorption Through Special Routes of Administration
   E. Distribution
   F. Metabolism
   G. Excretion
III. Toxicologic Testing Methodologies
   A. Acute Toxicity Studies
   B. Dermal Irritation, Sensitization, and Phototoxicity
   C. Eye Irritation
      Table 23–1. Numerical toxicity rating definitions

KEY POINTS

- Toxicology is the study of the mechanisms of action and adverse effects of chemical agents in living organisms. Toxicologists identify the nature of health damage that may be produced by a chemical substance and the range of doses over which damage is produced.
- Every known chemical, if present in sufficient amount, has the potential to produce injury or death.
- The amount needed to produce an adverse effect varies considerably among materials. Key elements in assessing the degree of human risk for any given chemical are the exposure, absorption, and metabolism of the substance. Toxic effects of a chemical agent in humans or animal models are not produced unless the agent or its metabolites reach appropriate receptors in the body at a concentration and for a length of time sufficient to initiate the toxic manifestations. The most important factors influencing this critical event are the route of contact of the agent, the dose, and the duration of exposure.
- The major routes by which toxic agents gain access to the body are by inhalation (through the lungs), absorption (through the skin), or ingestion (through the gastrointestinal tract). Another possible route of exposure is by parenteral administration (through injection). Most industrial exposure is by inhalation or dermal absorption.
- The amount of exposure is an important factor in the development of toxicity. Toxic manifestations usually occur with greater frequency and severity as the dose increases (the dose-response relationship). This dose-response relationship is not as relevant in situations where there is an immunologic reaction in the disease process.
- The time period over which exposure occurs is important in the manifestation of the toxic effect. In general, the adverse effect associated with a single dose is reduced when the total amount in the single dose is divided into two or more separately administered smaller doses.
- Factors that influence the concentration of toxic materials that reach a receptor site include the rate and amount of chemical absorbed; the distribution of the toxicant within the body; the rate of metabolism or biochemical transformation, if any; and the rate of excretion of the toxicant or its metabolites.
- After absorption, the distribution of a chemical toxicant occurs through the bloodstream. Distribution depends principally on the ability of the chemical to pass through the cell membranes of the various tissues of the body and the affinity of the various tissues for the chemical.
- Metabolism refers to the chemical transformation of compounds that can occur in an organism as a result of enzymatic reactions. The types of enzymatic reactions that can occur within an organism include catabolic or breakdown reactions of oxidation, reduction, and hydrolysis, and synthetic conjugation reactions.
- A number of factors influence the rate of biotransformation. These include differences in age, nutritional status, sex, species and strain of animal, and the presence of an underlying disease.
- Toxicants are primarily eliminated from the body through the kidney, but the liver and biliary systems, the lungs, sweat, tears, and even breast milk can all excrete chemicals from the body.

- Two fundamental assumptions underlie all animal toxicity testing: (1) effects produced by the compound in laboratory animals are often the same as the effects observed in humans; (2) the rate of adverse health effects increases as the dose or exposure increases.
- Acute animal toxicity studies are used to determine the median lethal dose for a chemical (LD_{50}).
- Subchronic exposure studies are used to evaluate and characterize the potential toxicity of a compound when administered to experimental animal on a daily basis over a period of 3 to 4 months.
- In vitro toxicology assays utilize cell cultures and bacterial systems outside the living animal. These assays provide a rapid and relatively inexpensive means of identifying mutagenicity and a material's ability to damage DNA. The most widely used bacterial test system for identifying mutagenicity is the *Salmonella typhimurium* microsome test commonly called the Ames assay.
- An understanding of toxicologic principles and testing methods can assist the physician in the evaluation of patients who have symptoms or illness that are possibly caused by an occupational exposure. A detailed occupational history helps assess the degree and nature of the individual's contact with toxic material. The Material Safety Data Sheet (MSDS), if available, can provide important information.

QUESTIONS

1. Which one of the following general principles, objectives, or statements is **incorrect?**

A. Toxicology is the study of mechanisms of action and adverse effects of chemicals in living organisms.
B. The main objective of toxicology is to identify the nature of health damage that may be produced by a chemical substance and the range of doses over which damage is produced.
C. Toxic effects are always produced when the chemical agent or its metabolite reaches appropriate receptors in the body.
D. If the absorption, distribution, metabolism, and excretion of a material are similar in humans and a particular animal species, test results in that species are generally predictive of toxicity of the material in humans.
E. Metabolism of foreign compounds can occur in the intestines, kidney, liver, and brain.

2. Which one of the following is **incorrect?**

A. The amount of gas that enters the blood from the alveoli does not depend on the solubility of the gas.
B. The stratum corneum is the primary anatomical barrier to dermal absorption.
C. The GI tract is an especially important route of absorption for environmental exposures.
D. The site of accumulation of a toxicant or its metabolite may or may not be the site of toxicologic activity.
E. The most common routes of exposure are inhalation, followed by dermal, followed by ingestion.

3. The extrapolation of animal testing to humans is dependent on two assumptions. One is that the toxic effects in animals are the same as in humans. The other is that the rate of adverse effects increases as the absorbed dose or exposure increases (dose-response). Which one of the following statements about animal toxicity tests is **incorrect?**

A. Acute toxicity tests can determine acute toxic effects as well as the concentration or dose likely to be lethal to 50% of animals, e.g., LD_{50} or LC_{50}.

B. Subchronic toxicity tests usually involve administering a test chemical to two species in a manner similar to that expected for humans. The duration of exposure is usually several months.

C. Chronic toxicity tests involve exposing the test animals to the test compound for their lifetime (usually at least 2 years). Observations suggesting carcinogenic effects include the types of neoplasms, an increased incidence of neoplasms, the occurrence of neoplasms earlier than in controls, and an increased multiplicity of neoplasms.

D. In vitro assays are slow and relatively expensive ways to determine mutagenicity.

E. Usually, but not always, a dose-response relationship exists for toxic materials.

4. *Which of the following factors influence whether a sufficient concentration of a toxic material reaches receptor sites within the body to initiate an adverse effect?*

A. The rate and amount of the material that is absorbed.
B. The distribution of the material within the body.
C. The rate of metabolism or biochemical transformation.
D. The rate of excretion of the toxicant or its metabolites.
E. All of the above.

5. *Which of the following sized particle are most likely to be deposited in the tracheobronchiolar regions of the lung after inhalation?*

A. Particles that are 10 μm or larger
B. Particles that are greater than 25 μm
C. Particles that are between 2 and 5 μm in size
D. Particles of 1 μm and below
E. None of the above

6. *The objective of subchronic exposure studies is to evaluate and characterize the potential toxicity of a compound when administered to experimental animals over which of the following time periods?*

A. A single occasion
B. Over 3 days
C. Over 20 days
D. Over 3 to 4 months
E. Over 24 to 30 months

$$\text{24}$$

Epidemiology and Biostatistics

OBJECTIVES

- State the characteristics of epidemiology that distinguish it from other perspectives
- Discuss the shortcomings of epidemiology
- Explain the characteristics of the major observational epidemiologic study designs
- Discuss the application of biostatistics in epidemiologic studies
- Discuss major factors that affect interpretation of epidemiologic studies, including causation

OUTLINE

    I. Strengths and Limitations of Epidemiology
   II. Observational Versus Experimental Studies
  III. Types of Observational Studies
       A. Cohort Study
          1. Advantages and Disadvantages
       B. Case-Control Study
          1. Advantages and Disadvantages
       C. Cross-Sectional Study
          1. Advantages and Disadvantages
  IV. Biostatistical Aspects of Epidemiologic Investigations
       A. Sample Size and Power
       B. Assessing Chance Variation
       C. Multiple Hypothesis Testing
       D. Analytic Techniques
          1. The 2×2 Table
          2. Cohort Methods
          3. The Standardized Mortality Ratio
          4. The Proportionate Mortality Ratio
   V. Interpretation of Epidemiologic Data
       A. Bias
       B. Confounding

KEY POINTS

- Epidemiology is the study of distribution and determinants of disease in human populations. The fundamental goal of these investigations is to obtain valid and reasonably precise estimates of exposure-disease associations in groups.
- Epidemiologic studies measure the risk of disease directly in human populations. There is no need to rely on questionable extrapolations across animal species to estimate the impact of an exposure in humans. It is possible in epidemiology to examine the consequences of an occupational or environmental exposure in the manner in which it actually occurs in humans, not the artificial manner in which laboratory studies of animals are done. The issues of dose, route of exposure, concomitant exposures, and host factors are also directly assessed.
- Shortcomings of the epidemiologic method include the following: (1) low-level risks are difficult to detect; (2) the long latency period of most chronic diseases make detection of exposure-disease associations quite difficult and render timely evaluation of new agents virtually impossible; (3) there are often many concurrent exposures, which can be difficult to disentangle; and (4) there is an inability to control for unknown confounding in the data.
- The most common type of study in occupational epidemiology is the cohort study, in which information on a factor (or factors) is collected in a defined population that is followed over time for the occurrence of a disease (or diseases). The disease rate among those exposed is compared to the rate among nonexposed to assess if there is an association between the study factor and disease.
- The prospective study takes a long time to complete, since investigators have to wait sometimes years before acquiring enough cases of disease (or death). A retrospective cohort study may be used to eliminate this long follow-up period. Past records of individuals are used to characterize the exposure status of the study subjects, and the disease status is determined until a particular date.
- The major methodologic advantage of the cohort design is that information on exposure is recorded before the development of disease. This eliminates recall bias.
- The case-control study examines two groups. One group consists of people with a particular disease and the other consists of those from the source population or study base without the disease. From each person in the two groups, information regarding past exposures and habits is obtained. If the exposure of interest is reported by a larger proportion of cases than controls, an association between the exposure and disease can be said to exist. Case control studies are more efficient and suitable for the study of rare diseases and diseases with long latency periods.
- In a cross-sectional study, people are selected regardless of exposure or disease status. Often this study design is called a survey or prevalence study.
- The number of subjects needed to assess the potential exposure-disease relationship is a fundamental issue when planning a study.
- The larger the sample size, the greater the power to detect a specified difference in risk. The power of a study is the probability of finding an association of a given magnitude between an exposure and a disease when, in fact, it exists.
- Chance variation refers to the natural variation in health outcomes observed among similarly exposed individuals. Two statistical tools used for assessing the role of chance are the p value and the confidence interval. The p value is the probability of obtaining by chance alone a difference in disease rates between the exposed and unexposed as large as or more extreme than what was observed. A p value of .005 means that the probability of obtaining by chance alone an exposure effect as large

as or more extreme than what was observed is only 5 per 1,000. Small *p* values (below .05) are sometimes referred to as statistically significant. The confidence interval gives the plausible values for the actual effect of exposure with a desired degree of confidence. For example, the 95% confidence interval for the risk associated with an occupational exposure is an interval in which the true relative risk will be included 95% of the time. A 95% confidence interval that includes 1.0 implies that a value of 1.0 for the relative risk is plausible and thus the null hypothesis of no exposure effect is consistent with the data.

- The simplest statistical technique, the 2×2 table, is useful when occupationally exposed and unexposed individuals are followed for equal amounts of time for disease incidence.
- The most commonly used epidemiologic method that accounts for variable follow-up is the calculation of the disease incidence rate. It is calculated by dividing the observed number of cases of disease by the total person-years of follow-up.
- Sometimes a study base or internal control group is not available. In these situations it is necessary to rely on external comparisons. The observed number of cases in an exposed cohort are compared to the expected number using a set of known, standard disease rates. This estimate of relative risk is called the standardized mortality ratio (SMR).
- Occasionally the only information available for assessing occupational risks consists of the death certificates from individuals employed in an industry. The proportionate mortality ratio (PMR) is useful for comparing the distributions of various causes of death based on the death certificate review.
- Bias or systematic error is usually a result of flaws in the study design or data collection. Confounding refers to the effect of an extraneous variable that may partially or completely account for an apparent association between a study exposure and disease.
- A set of criteria or principles has been developed that is used when confronted with a possible causal relationship between exposure and disease. These include the strength of association, the presence of a dose-response relationship, the time sequence between exposure and disease, the consistency of the report with other studies, and the biologic coherence.

QUESTIONS

*1. Which one of the following is **incorrect?***

A. Epidemiology is the study of the distribution and determinants of disease in human populations.
B. Unlike clinical or individual perspectives, epidemiology's perspectives are based on populations.
C. Case reports and case series can establish causal relationships between exposure and disease.
D. With epidemiology, there is no need to rely on extrapolations across species to estimate impact on humans.
E. In epidemiology, the exposures are more representative of the real world in comparison to the relatively artificial exposures to laboratory animals.

2. Which of the following is true of epidemiologic investigation?

A. Low-level risks are frequently detectible with such methodology.
B. Bias is the distortion of an exposure-disease association by an extraneous variable.
C. Short latency periods make detection of a risk factor difficult since temporal correlations may not be revealed.
D. Epidemiologists rely on questionable extrapolations across species to estimate exposure risk.

E. Many epidemiologic investigations rely on industrial hygiene measurements for exposure estimation.

3. *Which one of the following is **incorrect?***

A. In a prospective cohort study, information about an exposure (or other factors) is collected in at least two defined populations (a study group and a comparison group) at the beginning of the study, then the occurrence of disease in those populations are followed over time. The relative risk is a ratio—the incidence rate in the study group divided by the incidence rate in the comparison group.
B. In a retrospective cohort study, the disease status of the study and comparison groups are determined at the present time. Comparisons are based on past exposures. This type of study is rarely found in occupational literature.
C. Comparison groups in cohort studies may be external to the population under study. For example, the mortality rate from leukemia in a group of workers exposed to a specific agent could be compared to the mortality rate for leukemia in the U.S. population.
D. The main advantage of the cohort design is that information on exposure is recorded before the development of disease. As a result, the investigator knows that the exposure preceded development of the disease (it eliminates recall bias).
E. Major disadvantages of the prospective cohort design are related to its high cost and long duration of observation.

4. *Which one of the following is correct?*

A. On July 14, 1995, you administer an employment questionnaire and nerve conduction testing to 1,000 people at the state fair. You are interested in determining the relationships, if any, between median nerve conduction delay at the wrist and body mass index or wrist squareness. This is an example of a case-control study.
B. On July 14, 1995, you identify two populations for study. One population works in a foundry; the other in a hospital. You perform MRI studies of the lumbar spine for both groups on July 15, 1995 to compare the prevalence of herniated nucleus pulposus of the L5-S1 disk among the two groups. This is an example of a prospective cohort study.
C. On July 14, 1995, you start to collect pulmonary function test results among all patients presenting to your office. Two years later, you compare the work history of those with significant obstructive lung defects (FEV_1 <60% predicted) to those with FEV_1 >75%. This is an example of a retrospective cohort study.
D. On July 14, 1995, you identify a population of uranium miners in Colorado and a population of recreational professionals in Colorado. You verify that none in either population has lung cancer at the beginning of the study. You observe the development of lung cancer among the groups over the next 20 years, then compare the incidence rate of lung cancer in uranium miners to recreational professionals. This is an example of a cross-sectional study.
E. On July 14, 1895, your grandfather (a renowned physician in his day) administered a survey to all people living in his home town. He asked people to estimate hours spent riding in a saddle and whether they had symptomatic hemorrhoids in the past year. This is an example of a cross-sectional study.

5. *You are interested in comparing the incidence of carpal tunnel syndrome (CTS) among hospital workers to physicians. The relative risk of carpal tunnel syndrome among hospital employees is 2.7. The 95% confidence interval is 0.95–5.2. Which one of the following is correct?*

A. The power of a study is the probability of missing an association when one actually exists. This study had high power.

B. In this study, the null hypothesis would be: There is no difference in the incidence of CTS among hospital workers compared to physicians.
C. Since the confidence interval varies from 0.95 to 5.2, the *p* value for the statistical test is small (less than .05).
D. The proper conclusion is that the relative risk of CTS is significantly increased among hospital employees in comparison to physicians.
E. Since this study failed to reveal an association, the hypothesis is not worthy of further study.

6. *Which one of the following is **not** a key principle in interpreting an epidemiologic study?*

A. strength of the association
B. dose-response effect
C. duration of study
D. consistency
E. time sequence of risk factor in disease

REFERENCES

Doll R, Peto R. *The causes of cancer.* New York: Oxford University Press, 1981.
Fraumeni JF Jr, Hoover RN. Current views of epidemiologic methods. *Federal Register* Part II, March 14, 1985:58–64.
Hoover RN. Detection of environmental cancer hazards: Epidemiologic methods. *J. Med. Soc. N.J.* 75:746, 1978.
MacMahon B, Pugh TF. *Epidemiology: principles and methods.* Boston: Little, Brown, 1970.

25

Medical Surveillance

OBJECTIVES

- Explain the primary purpose of medical surveillance
- Identify factors used to assess the needs of a medical surveillance program
- List the five phases of effective screening programs
- Explain the attributes of each of the five phases associated with screening programs

OUTLINE

    I. Needs Assessment
        A. The Work Site
            Table 25–1. Phases of medical surveillance programs
            Table 25–2. Needs assessment
        B. Toxicity of Materials
   II. Selecting Programmatic Goals and Target Population
                 Table 25–3. Purposes of medical surveillance programs
        A. Screening for Occupational Disease
        B. Screening for Nonoccupational Disease
        C. Surveillance to Detect Exposure Rather Than Disease
        D. Baseline for Future Reference
        E. Risk Factor Identification
 III. Choosing Testing Modalities
        A. Questionnaires
        B. Physical Examinations
        C. Chest Radiography
        D. Pulmonary Function Testing
        E. Assessment of Exposure: Biologic Monitoring
        F. Cancer Risk Screening
        G. Data Type Should Guide Interpretation
 IV. Interpretation of Data to Benefit the Individual
        A. Nonspecific Testing (Such as Liver Function Testing)
   V. Intervention Based on Results

    VI. Identification of Overexposures and Disease Patterns
   VII. Interpretation of Data for the Benefit of Groups of Workers
  VIII. Communication of Results
    IX. Program Evaluation
     X. Examples of Medical Surveillance
       A. Example 1. A Well-Known Hazard with an Established OSHA Standard
       B. Example 2. A Relatively New Commercial Substance with Limited Toxicologic Data
    XI. Examples of Surveillance Targets
       A. Example 3. Exposure to Dusts
          1. Medical History
          2. Pulmonary Function Testing
          3. Chest Radiographs
       B. Example 4. Exposure to Metals
          1. Lead
          2. Mercury
          3. Arsenic
       C. Example 5. Exposure to Solvents
          Table 25–4. Possible uses of biologic monitoring to assess solvent exposure
       D. Example 6. Ergonomic Surveillance
   XII. References

KEY POINTS

- Medical surveillance is the systematic collection, analysis, and dissemination of disease data on groups of workers designed to detect early signs of work-related disease. The primary purpose of medical surveillance is to prevent disease.
- To assess the needs of a medical surveillance program, factors involving the work site, toxicity of materials, and program goals must be considered. Screening employees to identify work-related disease at an early stage involves a search for previously unrecognized disease or abnormal physiologic or pathologic conditions at a stage at which intervention can slow, halt, or reverse the progression of the disorder.
- In some settings, medical surveillance is designed to detect exposure rather than disease, such as following exposure to some heavy metals. Medical surveillance can also be used to determine a baseline with which future examinations are compared.
- Decisions about tests used for medical surveillance should be based on the relative toxicity of the substance, the extent of control measures, sampling results, work practices, and the usefulness of the tests themselves. Medical surveillance is not a substitute for primary control measures. The inclusion of unnecessary tests may lead to difficulties in assessing false-positive results, cause alarm among the well population, and needlessly increase health care costs.
- In biologic monitoring, tests are used to measure the extent of environmental exposures. A biologic specimen (e.g., blood, urine, exhaled air) is analyzed for the quantity of an environmental chemical or one of its metabolites to provide an estimate of a worker's chemical exposure. Biologic monitoring can be helpful in evaluating a hazardous exposure that a person may have experienced.
- In the occupational setting, a number of techniques have been attempted to screen for cancer. These include assessment of exposure to carcinogens, determination of oncogene activation, cytogenetic monitoring, immunologic studies for cell surface antigens, cytologic morphologic studies, and clinical testing methods. These tests, however, have not been shown to be effective in evaluating individual patients.
- Minor abnormalities of tests that may be normal variants or may be due to nonoccupational factors can be perplexing.

- The intensity of intervention for risk factors must be chosen based on the gravity of the disease and the ability of the intervention to be effective. The implications for worker's compensation and employer liability should be addressed. The reporting of some diagnoses may be mandatory. The physician's ethical responsibility to the worker must be the foremost consideration, and a physician (no matter in whose employ) must never withhold any information for fear of adverse effects on the employer.
- Analysis of aggregate data may reveal information that is useful for preventing occupational disease. There are several ways by which analysis of medical surveillance data can provide beneficial information to groups of workers, rather than just the person tested. These include investigation of the index case or case clusters, the recognition of temporal or geographic trends, and an association of clinical and laboratory results with exposure status. Medical surveillance analysis ideally includes observation of absence patterns that may represent an occupational hazard.
- Information about medical surveillance data may be directed to several targets: workers, management, worker representatives (e.g., unions), and government. Such results should be distributed in a timely manner and in an understandable fashion.
- Detection of a medical condition that makes work unsafe for the individual, the public, or co-workers cannot be ignored. Management is not entitled to specific medical information about an individual, but only the clinician's opinion about its implications.

QUESTIONS

*1. Which one of the following is **not** a principle of screening?*

A. The screening must be selective and geared to the population at risk.
B. The disease should be identified in its latent stage, not when symptoms appear.
C. The screening test is both valid and reliable.
D. Screening is a form of primary prevention.
E. Treatment should be both available and effective at a stage when the disease is detectable.

*2. Which one of the following statements about biologic monitoring is **incorrect?***

A. Biologic monitoring is, in general, the measurement of a chemical or its metabolite in a bodily fluid, e.g., blood lead.
B. In general, the presence of an industrial compound or its metabolite in a bodily fluid indicates that the person is overexposed to the substance at work, e.g., carboxyhemoglobin.
C. The blood or urinary level of a chemical does not necessarily imply a particular adverse health effect.
D. Biologic monitoring data are used to assess exposure, not make a clinical diagnosis.
E. One advantage of biologic monitoring over air monitoring is that the biologic monitoring result usually represents an integration of an individual's total exposure from all sources and by all routes.

*3. Which of the following is **least** characteristic of an effective screening program?*

A. Identification of preclinical diseases at a stage when effective treatment is available.
B. Identification of the disease when the symptoms are not yet disabling.
C. Lengthy lead time between detection by screening and manifestation of a disease such as lung cancer.

D.   Lack of false-positive test results
E.   Lack of false-negative test results.

4. *Which one of the following is **incorrect**?*

A.   OSHA's standard for lead is very specific about who should be in the program.
B.   Lead usually affects the central nervous system of children and the peripheral nervous system of adults.
C.   Lead inhibits hemoglobin synthesis, thus producing anemia.
D.   Lead affects the kidneys and gastrointestinal tract.
E.   A blood lead level >40 μm/100 ml proves lead poisoning in adults.

5. *Which is **not** true about medical surveillance?*

A.   It is primarily used to detect chemical poisoning in workers.
B.   Screening may be conducted for nonoccupational disorders.
C.   Programs usually require occupational medical expertise.
D.   Objectives should be defined before program initiation.
E.   It is primarily for prevention, not for treatment of existing disease.

REFERENCES

Baselt RC. *Biological monitoring methods for industrial chemicals.* Davis, CA: Biomedical, 1980.
Lauwerys RR. *Industrial chemical exposure: guidelines for biological monitoring.* Davis, CA: Biomedical, 1983.
Lowry LK. Biological exposure index as a complement to the TLV. *J. Occup. Med.* 28:578, 1986.
Monster AC. Biological monitoring of chlorinated hydrocarbon solvents. *J. Occup. Med.* 28:583, 1986.

26

Risk Assessment

OBJECTIVES

Explain how to apply risk assessment in a clinical situation
Define the terminology associated with risk assessment
State methods to calculate daily exposure by route
List the principles of risk assessment

OUTLINE

KEY POINTS

The workplace and the environment have always contained risks. Although accidents have traditionally been the most important risks, the vast number of chemicals now used in the workplace and found in the environment have increased the complexity of assessing risk. Risks associated with exposure to chemicals may be hidden and hard to detect. The effects of some chemicals may have long latent periods.

By understanding the elements of the risk assessment calculation, the practicing physician can appreciate those parameters that can increase or decrease risk and provide appropriate guidance to individuals exposed to a variety of occupational and environmental hazards.

The three-step approach to an individual risk assessment should include (1) an understanding of current and past exposure based on actual dose (if available); (2) modification of risk factors in the workplace (through counseling, personal protective equipment, and engineering controls); and (3) a reassessment of the risks to provide the worker with input for determining acceptability of the risk.

It is recognized that a physician rarely has either the information or the time to perform a calculation-based (quantitative) risk assessment. Even so, there are numerous uncertainties in the assumptions involved in risk assessment, thus making it, at best, a rough estimate.

A physician can use a table, such as Table 26–1, to explain the numerical results of a risk assessment to patients. This is based on comparing risks of death for one situation to the risk of death in another situation. The acceptability of a certain risk must be evaluated by the patient.

There are several strategies that can be used to reduce the risk related to a certain exposure. As shown in Table 26–2, some reduce the concentration of the chemical and some reduce duration of exposure (per day and lifetime). Personal hygiene, personal protective equipment, and work practices may contribute to reducing the current hazard.

Risk assessment is a statistical procedure employed by various regulatory agencies in an attempt to define an acceptable level of risk for exposure to a hazardous substance. The process uses scientific evidence from human (epidemiology) and animal studies to develop models to predict toxicity of various substances at low levels of exposure. Formulas for calculating daily exposure for different routes of absorption are listed in Table 26–3.

NOEL is an acronym used to indicate a level of exposure at which there is no observed effect level.

QUESTIONS

*1. Which one of the following statements about risk assessment is **incorrect?***

A. Risk assessment is a statistical procedure employed by various regulatory agencies to define an acceptable level of risk for exposure to a hazardous substance.

B. Risk assessment uses scientific evidence from human and animal studies to develop models to predict the toxicity of a substance at low levels.

C. Limitations of risk assessment include the reliability of the data, the accuracy of extrapolating results from animals to humans, and the legitimacy of assuming a linear relationship between low doses of a substance and adverse health effects.

D. Regulatory agencies, such as the EPA, generally assume that potential human carcinogens have a threshold of exposure below which no increased risk of cancer is predicted.

E. The classic dose-response curve is shaped like a sigmoid, i.e., there is a threshold for low-level exposures.

2. A worker is exposed to a volatile organic compound for 8 hours per day, 5 days per week. The work is characterized as moderate physical activity with a inspiratory rate of 2 m³ per hour. The airborne concentration is 150 mg per m³. You may assume 100% absorption. What is the daily exposure for this worker?

A. 150 mg

B. 300 mg

C. 300 mg/m^3
D. $1{,}200 \text{ mg/m}^3$
E. $2{,}400 \text{ mg}$

3. *What factors increase the risk of adverse health effects secondary to exposure to a hazard?*

A. Duration of exposure
B. Concentration of exposure
C. Body weight
D. Only A and B
E. A, B, and C

4. *For which route is occupational exposure the easiest to quantify?*

A. oral
B. dermal
C. inhalation
D. either A, B, or C when personal protection equipment is recommended
E. all routes combined

27

Searching the Occupational Medical Literature

OBJECTIVES

- Discuss information resources used to review the medical literature
- Explain how to access the public literature through a medical library or personal computer
- List strategies for searching the literature using Medical Subject Headings (MeSH)

OUTLINE

I. Medical Information Resources
   A. Medical Books and Reference Texts
   B. Medical Libraries
   C. The National Library of Medicine
   D. Electronic Databases
II. Search Strategies
   A. Searching Using MeSH
       Table 27–1. An example of the Medical Subject Headings Tree Structure
   B. Free-Text Searching
III. Case Histories
       Table 27–2. Search for cataracts in workers with occupational exposure to solvents
       Table 27–3. Search for Crohn's disease and liver disease in workers with occupational exposure to solvents
   A. Cataracts
   B. Liver Disease
IV. References

KEY POINTS

- An essential aspect of occupational health practice is awareness of new associations between exposures to various agents and the development of a variety of illnesses.

The retrieval of toxicologic information is crucial to the formulation of an opinion that may have wide-ranging ramifications.

- A large variety of medical information resources are available to assist in searching both primary and secondary sources in the medical literature, including books and reference texts, medical libraries together with research librarians, the National Library of Medicine (NLM), electronic databases, and a system for the classification of biomedical information by the NLM.
- The medical subject headings (MeSH) list is an evolving vocabulary system developed by the NLM to govern the classification and retrieval of biomedical information. It has three components: the annotated alphabetical list (with subjects arranged in alphabetical order), the tree structure (a subject-arranged listing of the over 14,000 terms from the annotated list), and the permutated headings (which serves as a thesaurus for the MeSH).
- A literature search usually refers to scientific articles or research reports; book chapters and other forms of information are also included in databases. Many databases exist throughout the world, and they constantly change. The MEDLINE, TOX-LINE, and TOXNET are basic to occupational medicine, but others may be helpful. The MEDLINE database is one of the most heavily used databases in the health care field.
- It is essential to have a sound strategy to logically search for information. This strategy should define the types of sources to retrieve.

QUESTIONS

1. The MEDLINE database file contains citations from the biomedical literature dating back to:

A. 1946
B. 1956
C. 1966
D. 1976
E. 1986

2. The MEDLINE file contains citations from which indexes?

A. Science Citation Index and Index Medicus
B. Index Medicus, International Nursing Index, and Index to Dental Literature
C. Toxicology Abstracts, Index Medicus, and Science Citation Index
D. Index Medicus, Nutrition Abstracts, and International Nursing Index
E. Index Medicus, Biological Abstracts, and Chemical Abstracts

3. An article abstract is:

A. the full text of an article.
B. the editor's review of the article.
C. the author's summary of the article.
D. the indexer's review of the article.
E. a peer review of the article.

28

Ergonomics

OBJECTIVES

- Explain the fundamental principles related to upper extremity ergonomics (epidemiology, physiology, and biomechanics)
- List the generic risk factors and recognize limitations to their application
- Discuss the fundamental principles related to low back ergonomics (epidemiology, psychophysics, physiology, and biomechanics)
- Explain the principles of the revised NIOSH guide and recognize its limitations

OUTLINE

I. Upper Extremity Disorders
  A. Epidemiologic Context
       Table 28–1. Number and type of disorders reported in previous studies of upper extremity morbidity
  B. A Physiologic Model—Localized Muscle Fatigue
       Figure 28–1. The Rohmert curve
       Figure 28–2. The Ergonomic Job Analysis Form used in Dr. Rodger's physiologic model
  C. A Biomechanical Model
       Figure 28–3. Sources of intrinsic compressive load on tendons and their sheaths
  D. Generic Risk Factors
       Table 28–2. Generic risk factors
    1. Force
    2. Posture
       Figure 28–4. Effects of posture on the worker
    3. Repetitiveness
    4. Use of Vibrating Tools
    5. Other Modifying Factors
    6. Localized Mechanical Compression
  E. Summary

II. Ergonomic Considerations in Low Back Pain
    A. Epidemiologic Context
    B. Biomechanical Models for Estimating Low Back Pain Risk Factors
        Figure 28–5. A lumbar motion segment: compression, tension, shear, and torsion
        Figure 28–6. Relationship between incidence rate of low back pain and disk compression
        Figure 28–7. Printout from the University of Michigan 2-Dimensional Static Strength Model
    C. Psychophysical Criteria for Low Back Pain
        Figure 28–8. The incidence and severity rates for musculoskeletal injuries with increasing strength demands
        Table 28–3. An excerpt from the maximum acceptable weight of lift tables
    D. Physiologic Model for Estimating Risk for Low Back Pain
    E. The NIOSH Guide/Equation for Manual Lifting
        Figure 28–9. Definition of distances used in the NIOSH guide for manual lifting
    F. Postural Stresses
    G. Summary
III. References

KEY POINTS

- The field of ergonomics is evolving. In some areas, knowledge is limited, but personal beliefs and opinions are prevalent.
- External sources of stress on a worker are called stressors. The effect of such stresses on or inside the worker's body is called strain.
- In clinical practice, physicians apply ergonomics when making decisions about work-relatedness of some musculoskeletal conditions and about return-to-work.
- Disorders of the upper extremity can be grouped into two large categories: disorders of the muscle-tendon units and disorders of the nervous system. Disorders of the muscle-tendon units include tenosynovitis, peritendinitis, and epicondylitis. Disorders of the nervous system include conditions such as carpel tunnel syndrome (CTS).
- In general, disorders of the muscle-tendon unit are much more common than CTS. When CTS is suspected to be related to work, there are almost always muscle-tendon unit disorders among patients or other workers performing the same job.
- The physiologic model for assessing upper extremity exposure is based on minimizing localized muscle fatigue—a reversible physiologic state.
- Concentric or sometric muscle actions, described in terms of their intensity, duration of action, and duration of recovery, are the most characteristic exertions related to localized muscle fatigue.
- The intensity of the exertion is expressed as a percent of maximal force. It is the required force divided by the worker's task— specific maximal force.
- Using Rohmert's work, it is possible to specify required recovery periods for exertions of known intensity (% maximal force) and duration of exertion. There is one job analysis model available that is based on these physiologic principles. The task variables are effort level, continuous effort time, and efforts per minute.
- The biomechanical model describes the responses of a muscle-tendon unit to stretching or compression. Stretching, or tensile loads, are described by their magnitude and duration of the applied force, duration of recovery, strain rate, and number of cycles.
- Compressive forces may be extrinsic (from outside the body) or intrinsic (inside the body). Intrinsic compression is related to a loaded tendon turning a corner. Intrinsic

compression can be estimated by knowing the intensity of the tensile load, the radius of curvature of the surface, and the length of arc of contact. These latter two are related to posture.

- The Strain Index is a semi-quantitative job analysis methodology based on six risk variables. These include intensity of exertion, duration of exertion, exertions per minute, hand/wrist posture, speed of work, and duration of task per day.
- Generic risk factors include force, posture, repetitiveness, use of vibrating tools, other modifying factors, and local mechanical compression. Of these, force is probably the most important. Several are interrelated.
- Low back pain is a common condition among adults in general, including working adults. Among workers, overexertion is the most common cause. The exact anatomic cause of low back pain is generally unknown. Disk degeneration is believed to play a role.
- The biomechanical models related to the lower back are primarily used to estimate compressive force on the lumbar intervertebral disks. At high levels of disk compression, cartilage end-plate fractures occur that, if accumulated, impair hydration of the disk and lead to a permanent loss of disk height. This is the beginning of disk degeneration.
- Psychophysical criteria refer to strength requirements in relation to strength capability. When requirements exceed capability, the worker is at risk for an overexertion injury. There are several ways to measure back or lifting strength: sometrics, isokinetics, maximum acceptable weight, etc. Maximum acceptable weight may be especially useful for job design.
- A physiologic model related to the lower back is called the energy expenditure model. It estimates the aerobic demand of a job that can be compared to consensus levels of acceptable aerobic demands.
- The NIOSH guide (or equation) for manual lifting is a job analysis tool that indicates disk composition, strength demands, and energy expenditure through one result. The recommended weight limit for a job or task is calculated by multiplying the numerical values of six task variables. These include multipliers for horizontal distance, vertical distance, travel distance, couplings, frequency of lift, and duration of lift.
- Postural stress is another risk factor for low back pain. It refers to prolonged awkward postures.

QUESTIONS

1. *What is known about the relationship between upper extremity disorders and work is derived from three disciplines: epidemiology, physiology, and biomechanics. Which one of the following statements regarding these disciplines is **incorrect**?*

A. Disorders of the muscle-tendon unit are more common than CTS.
B. In the physiologic model of localized muscle fatigue, force is characterized as percent maximal force. Percent maximum force is equal to the required force divided by the task-specific maximal force.
C. In the physiologic model, posture is an independent risk factor.
D. In the biomechanical model, posture is an independent risk factor.
E. The Strain Index is a biomechanical model that incorporates six task variables.

2. *Generic risk factors for upper extremity disorders include force, posture, repetitiveness, use of vibrating tools, and other modifying factors. Which one of the following is **incorrect** regarding upper extremity cumulative trauma disorders?*

A. The forcefulness of a task may be the most significant generic risk factor.

B. Posture may not be a primary risk factor. It may be important because of its effects on and interactions with force.
C. Nonneutral wrist postures are associated with increased intracarpal pressure. Since wrist braces inhibit nonneutral wrist postures, they should prevent the development of CTS.
D. Hand-held power tools are an important factor related to the risk of developing hand-arm vibration syndrome.
E. The temporal characteristics of the job tasks are important, but must be considered in the context of the forcefulness of the exertions.

3. *Our knowledge about the ergonomic factors associated with low back pain is more advanced than similar knowledge about the upper extremity. Which one of the following is* **incorrect?**

A. Disk degeneration is better considered a disease process where repeated episodes of high disk compression are believed to cause repeated cartilage end-plate fractures. Eventually, the end plates are sufficiently scarred to permanently impair hydration of the nucleus pulposus, thus initiating the degenerative process.
B. Whenever the strength requirements of the job exceed the corresponding strength capability of the worker, the worker is at risk of an overexertion injury.
C. Energy expenditure reflects the aerobic demands of the job. It can be estimated from tables or an energy expenditure model.
D. The revised NIOSH guide incorporates six task variables that are related to the lifting task. These six task variables include horizontal distance, vertical distance, travel distance, frequency, duration, and couplings.
E. Postural stresses are estimated by evaluating a person's posture during a dynamic lifting task.

4. *Which one of the following task variables is* **not** *relevant to the physiologic model for localized muscle fatigue?*

A. vibration
B. intensity of exertion (expressed as a percentage of maximal strength)
C. duration of exertion
D. duration of recovery
E. the posture used when performing the exertion

5. *Which one of the following mechanisms for low back pain is* **not** *included in the revised NIOSH guide?*

A. disk compression force
B. energy expenditure
C. strength requirements
D. vibration
E. only B and D above

REFERENCE

Simonson E. Introduction. In: Simonson E, ed. *Physiology of work capacity and fatigue.* Springfield, IL: Thomas, 1971:xi.

29

Molecular Genetics

OBJECTIVES

- Recall the principles and terminology of molecular genetics
- Explain the relationship between molecular genetics and genetic testing
- Discuss the basis and application of molecular genetic assays
- Explain the ethical, legal, and social implications related to the use of genetic testing, especially in the workplace

OUTLINE

KEY POINTS

- The genetic basis of disease and disease risk is the focus of many research laboratories, and is expected to have wide-ranging clinical importance. The lessons learned through molecular genetics will affect medical decision making, worker protection, risk assessment processes, and other areas of occupational medicine practice.

- Genetic testing might allow the physician to predict which workers are at risk for specific diseases, identify who needs additional workplace protection, and suggest maximal allowable exposures, ethical issues notwithstanding.

- It also may be useful for detection of an occupational etiology for a disease in a worker or provide prognostic information. The primary goal for biomarkers, however, is to prevent disease and secondarily for the early detection of disease.

- Molecular genetics is the study of genes and gene structure. There are more than 100,000 human genes located on 46 chromosomes. Exons are parts of genes that are transcribed; introns are parts that are not. The genetic language that codes for the amino acid sequence in proteins is organized in triplets called codons.

- Diversity in cellular functions and characteristics are controlled through variations in gene sequences. Any variation that occurs in more than 1% of the population is considered a polymorphism. It is estimated that genetic polymorphisms occur in approximately every 500 bases.

- Diseases in every organ and body system may be caused by genetic dysfunction due to point mutations, gene deletions, or gross chromosomal aberrations.

- Exogenous exposures such as viruses and chemicals may cause mutations in genes. Genetic dysfunction can also be acquired through endogenous mutational mechanisms such as oxidative damage by chemicals released from neutrophils, errors during cell replication, and others. In fact, endogenous mutations are estimated to occur millions of times each day in any one person but are efficiently repaired by the body.

- There are several recently developed genetic tests that can detect mutations, determine susceptibilities through genetic polymorphism detection, use biochemical methods to detect carcinogens bound to DNA, and measure abnormal or altered gene products and others. These include restriction enzyme analysis, the polymerase chain reaction, DNA probes, sequencing studies, DNA adduct detection, cytogenetic assays, and the detection of gene products and proteins. A method of detecting DNA damage that does not require cell culture and examination of chromosomes during mitosis is the detection of micronuclei.

- Most genetic assays are used in the research setting, but several studies have demonstrated how such research might be applied to the worker and his/her health.

QUESTIONS

1. A polymorphism is defined as an inheritable trait that occurs in at least what percentage of the population?

A. 0.1%
B. 1.0%
C. 5.0%
D. 10%
E. 50%

*2. The polymerase chain reaction (PCR) amplifies parts of a gene from very small amounts of DNA that can be analyzed for the detection of conditions for all of the following **except:***

A. organophosphate poisoning.
B. chronic myelogenous leukemia.
C. bladder cancer risk.
D. RAS oncogene mutations.
E. HIV infection.

3. *Micronuclei in white blood cells are:*

A. normal parts of the cell involved in the metabolism of chemicals.
B. markers of cell death from chemical exposure.
C. markers of carcinogen exposure.
D. markers of mutagen exposure.
E. markers of cells entering mitosis.

4. *Genetic testing might be used to:*

A. deny persons health or life insurance if they carry a marker of disease risk.
B. deny workers a job if they carry a marker of disease risk.
C. focus disease prevention strategies on persons who are at increased risk of a disease, allowing limited resources in education to be used for only those persons at risk.
D. revise risk assessments, calculating different risks for populations carrying different genetic traits.
E. all of the above.

REFERENCES

Blum M, et al. Molecular mechanism of slow acetylation of drugs and carcinogens in humans. *Proc. Natl. Acad. Sci. U.S.A.* 88:5237, 1991.

Heddle JA, et al. The induction of micronuclei as a measure of genotoxicity. A report of the U.S. Environmental Protection Agency Gene-Tox program. *Mutat. Res.* 123:61, 1983.

Hewlett IK, et al. Assessment by gene amplification and serological markers of transmission of HIV-1 from hemophiliacs to their sexual partners and secondarily to their children. *J. Acquir. Immune Defic. Syndr.* 3:714, 1990.

Kato N, et al. Detection of hepatitis C virus ribonucleic acid in the serum by amplification with polymerase chain reaction. *J. Clin. Invest.* 86:1764, 1990.

Kawajiri K, et al. Identification of genetically high risk individuals to lung cancer by DND polymorphisms of the cytochrome P450IA1 gene. *FEBS* 263:131, 1990.

Kurzrock R, et al. Molecular diagnostics of chronic myelogenous leukemia and Philadelphia-positive acute leukemia. In: Furth M, Greaves M, eds. *Cancer cells: molecular diagnostics of human cancer.* New York: Cold Spring Harbor Press, 1989:9–13.

Manos MM, et al. Cancer cells: molecular diagnostics of human cancer. In: Furth M, Greaves M, eds. *Cancer cells: molecular diagnostics of human cancer.* New York: Cold Spring Harbor Press, 1989:209–214.

30

Medical Center Occupational Health

OBJECTIVES

- List the major components of a medical center occupational health program
- Discuss common biologic hazards associated with a medical center
- Discuss common chemical hazards associated with a medical center
- Explain common physical hazards associated with a medical center
- Explain common psychosocial hazards associated with a medical center

OUTLINE

<pre>
   I. Medical Center Occupational Health Programs
      A. Hazard Assessment
      B. Hazard Control
      C. Medical Evaluation
  II. Biologic Hazards
      A. Blood-Borne Pathogens
      B. Other Infectious Agents
      C. Latex Allergy
      D. Tuberculosis
         Table 30–1. Summary of important recommendations and work restrictions
             for personnel with infectious diseases
      E. Laboratory Animal Allergy
      F. Hazardous Waste Disposal
 III. Chemical Hazards
      A. Waste Anesthetic Gases
      B. Antineoplastic Agents
      C. Sterilants
      D. Disinfectants
      E. Laboratory Safety
  IV. Physical Hazards
</pre>

        A. Exertion
        B. Heat
        C. Noise
        D. Radiation
        E. Lasers
        F. Indoor Air Quality
    V. Psychosocial Hazards
        A. Stress
        B. Chemical Dependency
   VI. Conclusion
  VII. References
 VIII. Appendix to Chapter 30: Occupational Hazards by Location in the Hospital

KEY POINTS

- Medical centers are complex workplace environments that pose an assortment of safety and health hazards for workers. This includes biologic, chemical, physical, and psychosocial hazards. Medical center occupational health programs can be influenced by a variety of regulatory agencies, including the Occupational Safety and Health Administration (OSHA), the Food and Drug Administration (FDA), the Nuclear Regulatory Agency (NRC), the Joint Commission on Accreditation of Health Care Organizations (JCAHCO), and others.
- Every medical center should establish and maintain a comprehensive occupational health and safety program. Physical inspection of the work site should be performed on a regularly scheduled basis by those capable of recognizing safety and health hazards.
- Foremost among biologic hazards are those associated with hepatitis B virus (HBV) and human immunodeficiency virus (HIV).
- The Blood-Borne Pathogens Standard requires that employees with occupational exposure to blood or other potentially infectious material be protected through a variety of measures as specified in a written exposure control plan.
- Some virus infections pose a teratogenic risk for pregnant employees. These include rubella, cytomegalovirus, and varicella zoster infections.
- An increasing number of complaints of latex allergy has been reported as the use of latex gloves has escalated. Allergic contact dermatitis involving the hands is the most common manifestation of latex allergy, but systemic reactions such as asthma or anaphylaxis can also occur.
- An increase in tuberculosis has been noted since 1985, and has been attributed to the HIV epidemic, inadequacies in the public health infrastructure for monitoring compliance with outpatient treatment, immigration from countries with a high TB prevalence, homelessness, and limited access to medical care. Of particular concern is the emergence of strains that are resistant to multiple antibiotics.
- The use of laboratory animals in large medical centers poses unique risks from allergy and zoonoses.
- Large amounts of medical waste pose problems related to disposal. This material may be infectious or may include noninfectious items that are otherwise hazardous (such as radioactive material or chemical items, some of which may be flammable or explosive).
- Adverse health effects can occur from exposure to trace levels of waste anesthetic gases in operating and recovery rooms, labor and delivery suites, and emergency areas and outpatient clinics.
- Antineoplastic agents can produce both acute and chronic health effects in health care workers who handle such agents.
- Chemical sterilants, such as ethylene oxide and formaldehyde, and a variety of disinfectants are also recognized as causes of health problems.

- Physical exertion is responsible for a high frequency of acute and chronic back pain complaints among health care workers. Other physical agents that may produce health problems include heat stress (in laundries, kitchens, and boiler rooms), noise exposure, radiation, and the use of lasers.
- Stress disorders are common among health care workers. In addition, chemical dependency is higher among this group than in the general population.

QUESTIONS

*1. Which one of the following is **incorrect** regarding biologic hazards in a medical center?*

A. OSHA's Blood-Borne Pathogens Standard specifically targets the prevention of hepatitis B virus (HBV) and human immunodeficiency virus (HIV) infection in health care workers.
B. Effective immunization programs for health care workers can help to prevent adverse reproductive outcomes.
C. A suspicion of latex allergy can be assessed by measurement of immunoglobulin E (IgE) antibodies or radioallergosorbent test (RAST).
D. A major component of a tuberculosis control program is the TB skin test.
E. OSHA has no standards for biologic hazards for health care workers.

2. Which one of the following is most correct regarding chemical and physical hazards in a medical center?

A. Exposure of operating room personnel to waste anesthetic gases is readily controlled by use of proper respirators.
B. Since the duration and degree of exposure to antineoplastic agents are short and relatively low, medical surveillance is not indicated.
C. Good work practice is the most efficient way to control ethylene oxide exposure.
D. Manual lifting, especially of patients, may be a significant hazard to some medical center employees.
E. The therapeutic applications of lasers pose a minimal threat to worker health.

*3. Which of the following is **incorrect** regarding medical center occupational programs?*

A. Hazard assessment is an important step in program development.
B. Hazard assessment involves physical inspection of both patient care and non–patient care areas.
C. Monitoring of airborne contaminants is usually not necessary.
D. Hazard control strategies include engineering controls, work practice controls, and personal protective equipment.
E. Certain workers need to be periodically evaluated as part of a medical surveillance program.

4. Which of the following is correct?

A. Every medical center should develop a TB exposure control plan based on traditional principles of TB control.
B. Employees who have previously had a positive TB skin test should receive a skin test at time of hire and at least at 12-month intervals.
C. Employees with a history of negative skin test results should not be skin tested.
D. People who have been immunized with BCG should not be skin tested.
E. TB skin testing should not be done more frequently than once per year.

*5. Which of the following is **incorrect** regarding medical center labs?*

A. Every laboratory should develop a safety policy and procedures.
B. Safety policies and procedures should emphasize staff training, container labeling, and ready employee access to Material Safety Data Sheets.
C. The management of physical hazards includes the development of procedures for safe handling of glassware and radionuclides.
D. The availability and use of personal protective equipment should be discouraged.
E. Medical center laboratories may be subject to OSHA's Laboratory Standard.

REFERENCES

CDC. Guidelines for preventing the transmission of tuberculosis in health-care settings with special focus on HIV-related issues. *M.M.W.R.* 39:17, 1990.
Klein BP, et al. Assessment of worker's compensation claims for back strains/pains. *J. Occup. Med.* 26:443, 1984.
OSHA. Bloodborne pathogens. 29 CFR 1910.1030.

Section 3 Answers

CHAPTER 21 ANSWERS

1. The answer is B. (Reference: p. 301)

The Bureau of Labor Statistics (BLS) of the U.S. Department of Labor reports statistics based on surveys of private companies with greater than 11 employees, excluding the self-employed, farmers, and government employees. The BLS showed that work-related illnesses and injuries in the United States increased by about 177,000 to nearly 6.8 million in 1990 (Bureau of Labor Statistics, 1991). The survey found nearly 332,000 new cases of occupational illness in 1990, with nearly 60% of these cases associated with repetitive motions such as vibrations and repeated pressure.

2. The answer is D. (Reference: p. 302)

One obstacle to physicians' recognition of job-related health problems is insufficient education. A survey in 1983 showed that 50% of medical schools taught courses in occupational health, but the average curriculum time was only 4 hours (Levy, 1985).

Another impediment to the recognition of work-related illness is a lack of uniqueness in the clinical manifestations of many occupational illnesses.

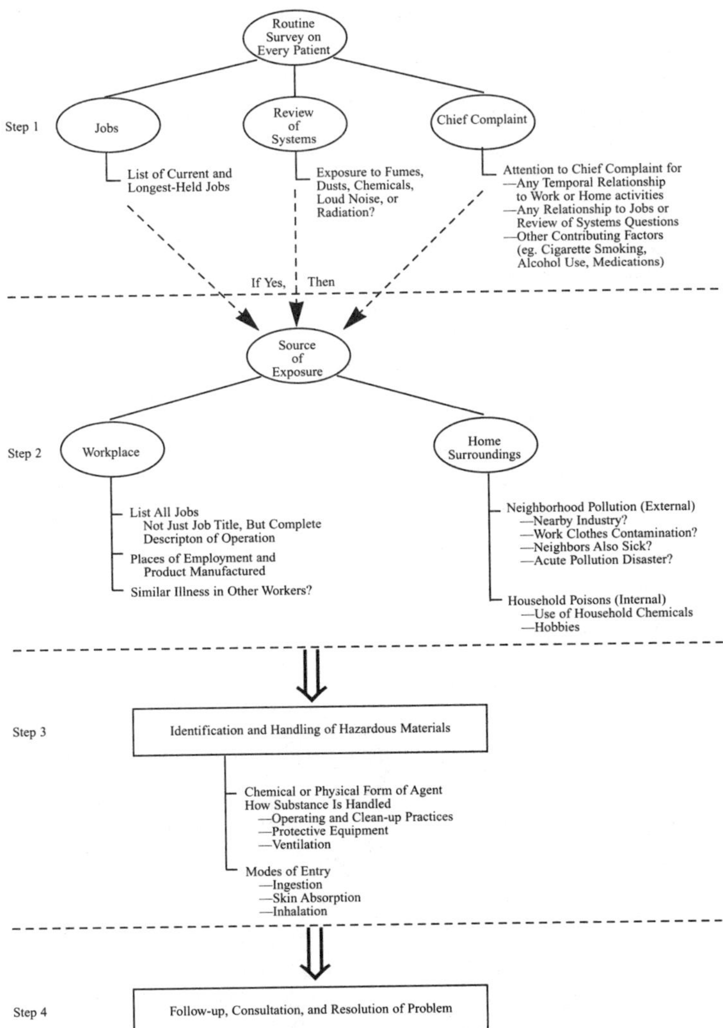

Figure 21-1. Systematic approach to history taking and diagnosis of occupational or environmental illness. (From R. H. Goldman and J. M. Peters. The occupational and environmental health history. *J.A.M.A.* 246:2831. Copyright 1981, American Medical Association.)

A long latency, or the period from initial exposure to presentation of disease, also leads to underrecognition of some occupational diseases.

3. The answer is A. (Reference: Figure 21–1, p. 304)

4. The answer is C. (See Figure 21–1)

5. The answer is A. (See Figure 21–1)

CHAPTER 22 ANSWERS

1. The answer is C. (Reference: pp. 321, 322)

The profession of industrial hygiene has as its main goals the recognition, evaluation, and control of workplace health hazards. Recognition of a hazard requires knowledge of both the processes and the hazards of the materials used in the processes. A thorough grasp of these matters is essential as the foundation for a health hazard investigation. Reviewing the various hazardous materials used will reveal potential air contaminants. In addition, reviewing the process can also uncover air contaminants that may be released as an intermediate or as a decomposition product in the chemical reaction. The decomposition products, at times, may be more hazardous than the raw materials.

After the type of air contaminant that may be released is determined, a sampling strategy can be developed that provides the information needed to evaluate the hazards.

This approach determines whether the person is overexposed to any air contaminants and by how much.

If an overexposure exists or if there is a desire to reduce employee exposure, a control measure is then determined to bring the air contaminant concentration below the exposure guideline or to the desired level. Control can be implemented by controlling the contaminant at the source, the pathway, or the person.

2. The answer is D. (Reference: pp. 322, 323)

Gases are substances that are normally in the gaseous state at room temperature; in contrast, vapors are the gaseous state of substances that are normally in the liquid state at room temperature.

A fume is a solid that has been vaporized and subsequently condenses. In the process of welding steel, for example, iron oxide fume is produced.

A mist is a liquid that has been dispersed into the air as fine droplets.

3. The answer is D. (Reference: pp. 322–325)

Monitoring employee exposure to air contaminants is the most visible aspect of the industrial hygienist's job. After the sampling strategy is determined, monitoring is performed to assess the extent of exposure to an air contaminant. Monitoring can be done by obtaining personal or area samples. In personal sampling, the sampling device or equipment, or both, is placed on the worker to ensure the most accurate exposure determination. For area sampling, the sampling apparatus is placed in the vicinity of the worker performing the job.

Organic gases and vapors can usually be collected with an absorbing material, like activated charcoal or silica gal. The absorbing material is contained in a small glass tube that is attached to a sampling pump, which draws a known volume of air.

Gases and vapors are usually reported in parts per million (ppm) units, a volume per volume measurement.

Dusts, including asbestos, coal, wood, and silica, can be monitored using a variety of instruments. The method used will depend on the type of dust, the size of the dust, the PEL or TLV, and the cost of the method. The most common method is to collect the dust on a preweighed filter medium using an air sampling pump.

The type of dust may determine the sampling method. Asbestos, for example, can be sampled with the filter method mentioned above. The filter medium is not weighed, however, as it is for nuisance dusts, but undergoes a microscopic analysis to determine the fiber count, rather than weight.

Respirable dusts, those of 10 μm or less in size, are monitored differently. In addition to an air sampling pump, a cyclone is used to separate the respirable from the larger dusts. This method is used to monitor respirable dusts such as silica that affect the terminal parts of the lungs.

Table 22–1. *Recognized exposure guidelines*

ACGIH threshold limit values (TLVs)
ACGIH biological exposure indices (BEI)
American Industrial Hygiene Association (AIHA) workplace environment exposure limit (WEEL)
National Institute for Occupational Safety and Health (NIOSH) recommended exposure limits (REL)
OSHA permissible exposure limits (PEL)

4. The answer is C. (Reference: Table 22–1, p. 327)

5. The answer is D. (Reference: p. 321)

The industrial hygienist, in particular, can offer valuable assistance to the physician who is asked to consider the health risks associated with certain work settings. The industrial hygienist, usually a graduate-level professional, can help in many areas, but most often in the following:
1. Determining the need for medical surveillance or special examinations of workers exposed to particular materials
2. Evaluating whether exposure to an occupational or environmental hazard may have contributed to the development of an occupational illness
3. Determining the presence of potential offending agents and the adequacy of ventilation systems in outbreaks of illness, such as indoor air pollution
4. Complementing the efforts of a physician who has completed a preliminary plant walk-through

6. The answer is E. (Reference: p. 322)

Any of these methods will control or limit the exposure because the contaminant does not reach the person or its concentration is reduced. Ideally, the most desirable approach would be to eliminate the hazard altogether, for example, by replacing the material with a nonhazardous material. Controlling the hazard at the person by using respiratory protection is the least desirable approach because it is dependent on the person's work habits. An enclosure, however, is desirable because it is independent of the worker's habits.

7. The answer is A. (Reference: p. 328)

The Biologic Exposure Indices (BEI), also published by the ACGIH, are warning levels of biologic response to a chemical or its metabolite. These values may be of use to a physician in determining a dose to a worker because other routes of entry, besides inhalation, may be involved. For example, blood lead analysis reflects the relative dose that the worker receives from all routes of exposure, including ingestion.

All guidelines refer to airborne exposures except for the Biologic Exposure Indices, which refer to safe biologic levels of the substance or its metabolite in body fluids or in expired air. Exposure guidelines can suggest to the occupational health professional how bad or good, in simplistic terms, a workplace exposure is. The TLVs developed by the ACGIH are updated annually and are meant to protect nearly all workers from adverse effects when they are repeatedly exposed to an agent.

CHAPTER 23 ANSWERS

1. The answer is C. (Reference: p. 333)

Toxicology is the study of the mechanisms of action and adverse effects of chemical agents in living organisms. The main objective of toxicology is to identify the nature of health damage that may be produced by a chemical substance and the range of doses over which damage is produced.

Measuring the effects of a chemical exposure directly in humans either through epidemiologic or controlled clinical studies provides the best evidence of a chemical's toxicity in humans. However, in most instances, it is impossible to study toxic effects in humans directly, and indirect methods such as toxicologic testing in animals and cell systems are necessary.

The underlying premise is that the final reaction of the chemical or its metabolite on the target cell within the animal or cell model is the same as that in humans.

2. The answer is A. (Reference: p. 335)

The amount of gas that enters the blood from the alveoli is dependent on the solubility of the gas in the blood. Highly soluble gases such as chloroform are rapidly taken up by the blood. A relatively large amount must be absorbed before the blood becomes saturated with the material and before a steady state or equilibrium is established, after which further net absorption from the lung does not occur. If the gas also has high lipid solubility, gas from the blood will rapidly enter body fat, and the time required to reach an equilibrium will be substantially longer.

3. The answer is D. (Reference: pp. 341, 342)

With appropriate modifications, the basic subchronic test can be used to evaluate mutagenesis, teratogenesis, and effects on reproductive capacity. Except for carcinogenesis and some forms of cytotoxicity, the subchronic test will usually reveal most forms of toxicity to adult animals.

In vitro toxicology assays utilize cell cultures and bacterial systems outside the living animal. These assays provide a rapid and relatively inexpensive means of identifying mutagenicity and a material's ability to damage DNA. Mutagenesis is the ability of chemicals to cause changes in the genetic material in the nucleus of cells in ways that can be transmitted during cell division.

4. The answer is E. (Reference: p. 334)

Several factors influence whether a sufficient concentration of a toxic material reaches receptor sites within the body to initiate an adverse effect. These include the rate and amount of the material absorbed; the distribution of the toxicant within the body; the rate of metabolism or biochemical transformation, if any; and the rate of excretion of the toxicant or its metabolites.

5. The answer is C. (Reference: p. 335)

For particulate matter and fogs or sprays of fine liquid droplets, the deposition within the pulmonary system depends to a great extent on the size of the particles. Particles of 5 μm or larger are usually deposited in the nasopharyngeal region and are carried by the mucous blanket of the ciliated nasal surface to the upper pharynx and eventually swallowed. Particles of 2 to 5 μm are deposited in the tracheobronchiolar regions of the lung, where they are rapidly and efficiently cleared by the upward movement of the mucous layer in the ciliated portions of the respiratory tract. Particles of 1 μm and smaller are able to reach the alveolar epithelium of the lung. In the alveoli, they may be absorbed into the blood or removed by two major routes: phagocytosis by phagocytes or macrophages, or removal through the lymphatic system.

6. The answer is D. (Reference: p. 341)

The objective subchronic exposure studies is to evaluate and characterize the potential toxicity of a compound when administered to experimental animals on a daily basis over a period of 3 to 4 months.

CHAPTER 24 ANSWERS

1. The answer is C. (Reference: p. 346)

Case reports and other forms of anecdotal data may alert an investigator to potential health risks, but the epidemiologic approach provides a systematic method for identifying and quantifying such health risks.

2. The answer is E. (Reference: p. 346)

Although epidemiology may be the only direct way to evaluate harmful or potentially harmful exposures in humans, the method has several shortcomings (Doll and Peto, 1981; Fraumeni and Hoover, 1985; Hoover, 1978; MacMahon and Pugh, 1970). Low-level risks are difficult to detect using this method. Very small increases in risk of exposed compared with unexposed groups may be accounted for in epidemiologic studies by bias (systematic error), confounding (distortion of exposure-disease association by an extraneous variable), or by chance.

The long latency (time from exposure to disease) of most chronic diseases is another obstacle in epidemiologic research.

Experimental studies have the distinct advantage of randomization, a procedure that distributes both known and unknown confounders equally between the test and control groups.

3. The answer is B. (Reference: p. 347)

To eliminate a possible 10- to 20-year follow-up period, a variant of the prospective cohort study has been developed, the retrospective cohort study. In a retrospective cohort study, the past records of individuals are used to characterize the exposure status of the study subjects, and the disease status (usually measured by mortality) is determined until the present (or until a particular date in the recent past). It is this variant that is most commonly found in the occupational literature, since the need to wait for a long follow-up period is eliminated, as it is already part of the design.

4. The answer is E. (Reference: p. 349)

In a cross-sectional study design, people are selected regardless of exposure or disease status. Often this study design is called a survey or prevalence study. Usually cross-sectional studies use random or probability sampling procedures to select subjects. This allows for the examination of the prevalence of a disease in a representative sample of the population, and analysis by various combinations of age, sex, and the presence or absence of disease is obtained at the same time, usually by interview.

5. The answer is B. (Reference: p. 350)

Two statistical tools for assessing the role of change are the p value and the confidence interval. P value is the probability of obtaining by chance alone a difference in disease rates between the exposed and unexposed as large as or more extreme than what was observed, assuming the null hypothesis, that is, that the exposure has no effect on disease incidence rates and that differences in disease rates are due solely to natural variation.

6. The answer is C. (Reference: p. 356)

Key principles in interpreting epidemiologic studies:
1. Strength of the association. In general, the higher the risk estimate, the less likely the finding is a result of confounding or bias.

2. Dose-response effect. If the risk of the disease rises with increasing exposure, a causal interpretation of the association is more plausible.
3. Time sequence. The exposure or risk factor must precede the disease.
4. Consistency. Results from other epidemiologic studies of the exposure-disease association should be similar.
5. Biologic coherence. Does the exposure-disease association make biologic sense given what is known of the natural history of the disease?

CHAPTER 25 ANSWERS

1. The answer is D. (Reference: p. 360)

Screening is considered a secondary preventive measure in the control of occupational illness, since the primary control measure is to reduce the hazardous exposure. Screening is based on a number of principles, including the following:

1. The screening test must be selective and geared to the population at risk.
2. The disease should be identified in its latent stage, not when symptoms appear.
3. Adequate follow-up study is necessary.
4. The screening test is both valid and reliable.
5. Benefits outweigh the costs and, where feasible, tests are noninvasive.
6. Treatment should be both available and effective at a stage when the disease is detectable.

2. The answer is B. (Reference: p. 362)

In biologic monitoring, tests are used to measure the extent of environmental exposures (Baselt, 1980; Lauwerys, 1983; Lowry, 1986; Monster, 1986). A biologic specimen (e.g., blood, urine, exhaled air) is analyzed for the quantity of an environmental chemical or one of its metabolites to provide an estimate of the worker's chemical exposure. Mere detection of a chemical, however, does not imply the presence of a disease or of toxicity.

3. The answer is D. (Reference: p. 360)

Screening is the search for a previously unrecognized disease or abnormal physiologic or pathologic condition at a stage at which intervention can slow, halt, or reverse the progression of the disorder. An effective screening program should identify disease at a stage at which intervention really matters.

4. The answer is E. (Reference: p. 371)

Detection of blood lead levels above 40 g/100 ml in itself does not prove that clinical toxic effects are present but does indicate that significant overexposure has occurred.

5. The answer is A. (Reference: p. 361)

Medical surveillance is not limited to screening (in which the participant will on the average benefit). In some settings, however, medical surveillance is designed to detect exposure rather than disease. For example, biologic monitoring (discussed later) measures concentrations of chemical agents or their metabolites in biologic specimens. This type of testing may be useful for determining if exposure is occurring even at levels that do not imply the presence of disease.

CHAPTER 26 ANSWERS

1. The answer is D. (Reference: p. 379)

Risk assessment is a statistical procedure employed by various regulatory agencies in an attempt to define an acceptable level of risk for exposure to a hazardous substance. Risk assessment uses available scientific evidence from human (epidemiology) and animal studies to develop models to predict toxicity of the various substances at low levels of exposure. Limitations inherent in this process include the reliability of the data, the accuracy of extrapolating results from animals to humans, and the legitimacy of assuming a linear relationship between low doses of a substance and the adverse health effect. This last problem manifests itself primarily in the evaluation of carcinogenic substances using information generated by U.S. governmental agencies, which do not recognize the presence of a threshold dose below which exposure to a substance is not a health risk.

2. The answer is E. (Reference: p. 380, Figure 26–3)

To perform relevant measurements and estimate an exposure, it is first necessary to assess the routes and conditions by which a worker may be exposed. Such exposure scenarios are usually specific to an absorption route, which may be oral, dermal, or inhalation. Inhalation estimates are the easiest to perform; by knowing the airborne level, one can calculate the exposure, as shown in Fig. 26–3. The air concentration is usually measured in milligrams or micrograms per cubic meter (mg/m^3 or $\mu g/m^3$). For the respiratory route, it is often assumed that there is total absorption of the inspired toxic vapors, although this is not the case for most substances. For an adult, air is inhaled at a rate of 1 m^3 per hour at rest and 2 m^3 per hour for moderately vigorous activity. An exposure estimate (dose) can be calculated by simply taking the product of the measured concentration and the air volume inhaled over a specified time interval.

```
Inhalation:

Daily exposure   =   air level   X    1-2m³   X   hours
                                      ─────        ─────
                                      hour          day


Oral (Soil):

Daily exposure   =   soil level   X   25 mg soil/day   X   % absorption


Dermal (Surfaces):

Daily exposure   =   surface level   X   1500 cm²   X

                     fraction of day exposed   X   % absorption

(The simplifying assumption of concentration equivalence between
of one-half the area of the arms and environment surface levels
will generally lead to an overestimation of exposure.)


All Routes:

Lifetime Average Daily Dose   =

        Daily exposure X days exposure/year   X   years exposure
        ──────────────────────────────────────────────────────────
              25,550 days/lifetime   X   70 kg
```

Figure 26–3. Formulas for calculating daily exposure by route. See text for explanation of terms.

3. The answer is E. (Reference: Table 26–2)

4. The answer is C. (Reference: p. 380)

To perform relevant measurements and estimate an exposure, it is first necessary to assess the routes and conditions by which a worker may be exposed. Such exposure scenarios are usually specific to an absorption route, which may be oral, dermal, or inhalation. Inhalation estimates are the easiest to perform.

Table 26-2. *Exposure factors that proportionally increase the calculated risk of cancer, assuming a linear-at-low-dose relationship.*

For all routes
    Years of exposure
    Hours of exposure per day
    Concentration of toxic substance[a]
For dermal exposure
    Surface area of skin exposed[a]
    Length of time substance remains on skin[b]
For oral exposure
    Mouthing episodes from contaminated hands, cigarettes, food, etc.[b]

[a]Reduced by personal protective equipment and work practices
[b]Reduced by hygiene

CHAPTER 27 ANSWERS

1. The answer is C. (Reference: p. 776, Appendix E)

MEDLINE is a heavily used biomedical database that may be accessed through many formats; it covers more than 4,000 journals from around the world. Indexing is based on MeSH. Citations contained in Index to Dental Literature, International Nursing Index, and Index Medicus are found in MEDLINE. Coverage begins with 1966 and continues to the present. Over 250,000 records are added each year.

2. The answer is B. (See above)

3. The answer is C. (Reference: p. 384)

Secondary sources include abstracts, which may take two forms: descriptive, indicating what has been done, and analytical, in which interpretations regarding data are presented. Review articles, another secondary source, attempt to summarize existing knowledge into a concise, compact form. The well-written review article identifies existing knowledge gaps within a subject and provides an extensive bibliography on the subject. It is an excellent starting point for becoming familiar with a topic.

CHAPTER 28 ANSWERS

1. The answer is C. (Reference: p. 398)

The physiologic model for assessment of upper-extremity exposures emphasizes minimizing localized muscle fatigue. Simonson (1971) defined fatigue as the transient loss of work capacity resulting from preceding work. Localized muscle fatigue is a reversible physiologic state. Its exact cause is unknown, but may involve accumulation of waste products, depletion of energy reserves, or hypoxemia secondary to impaired blood flow into the contracted muscle (Simonson, 1971). Symptoms of localized muscle fatigue may include a sensation of exhaustion, discomfort, or fatigue; increased perceived exertion; decreased strength; and loss of neuromuscular control.

2. The answer is C. (Reference: p. 405)

Physicians often recommend wrist braces at night, which minimize symptoms; that is, the braces prevent assuming extreme wrist postures during sleep so that the carpal canal pressure is kept below the ischemia threshold. Preventing the symptoms of CTS is quite different from preventing the development of carpal tunnel syndrome. The indiscriminate use of wrist braces during work, especially when the work is associated with dextrous use of the wrist and hand as opposed to the extremes of wrist posture reported in the literature, may actually aggravate the problem.

3. The answer is E. (Reference: pp. 414, 415)

A fourth risk factor for low back pain, not previously addressed, is static postural stresses, which refer to prolonged awkward postures, such as bending over for several minutes to perform a task that is at or below knee height. These kinds of static work postures are associated with static muscular work, thus leading to localized muscle fatigue of the support structures of the spine.

4. The answer is A. (See Answer 28–1)

5. The answer is D. (Reference: p. 413)

Before 1981, exposure assessment of manual handling tasks involved the estimation of (1) disk forces and static strength demands based on the two-dimensional model, (2) strength demands in comparison to maximum acceptable weights using the Liberty Mutual tables, and (3) energy expenditure demands of the job using either standardized tables or the energy expenditure model.

CHAPTER 29 ANSWERS

1. The answer is B. (Reference: p. 420)

Genes are the basic building blocks of heredity and control diverse body cellular functions and characteristics such as hair color, height, and facial features. This diversity is controlled through variations in DNA sequence. Any variation that occurs in more than 1% of the population is considered a polymorphism.

2. The answer is A. (Reference: pp. 419–420)

There are many applications for PCR. It is being used directly without other techniques for diagnosing viral infections (e.g., human immunodeficiency virus in lymphocytes (Hewlett, 1990), hepatitis B virus in liver and serum (Kato et al., 1990), and papilloma virus in uterine cervix (Manos et al., 1989)). It can be used to amplify mutated and structurally altered regions of a given gene (e.g., translocation of chromosomes by determining the breakpoint cluster region for the *bcr-abl* oncogene for the diagnosis of chronic myelogenous leukemia (Kurzrock et al., 1989)). Other applications involve the identification of single base mutations or genetic polymorphisms by designing primers that anneal only if matched to the unique sequence (e.g., oligospecific PCR for the identification of polymorphisms in the *N*-acetyltransferase gene predictive of cancer risk in workers exposed to aromatic amines (Blum et al., 1991)). PCR also is combined with other techniques whereby PCR amplification products can be subjected to restriction enzyme digestion to identify genetic polymorphisms or mutations (e.g., RFLP analysis for cytochrome P-450 genetic polymorphisms (Kawajiri et al., 1990)) or used for hybridization with mutation-specific probes (e.g., oligonucleotide hybridization for the detection of *ras* mutations).

3. The answer is D. (Reference: p. 423)

A method of detecting DNA damage that does not require cell culture and examination of chromosomes during mitosis is the detection of micronuclei (Heddle et al., 1983). Small chromosomal fragments are sometimes found to exist outside the nucleus. This assay is rapid, relatively inexpensive, and quantitative, so that its potential is greater as a screening test in humans for mutagenic exposures. It can be used for white blood cells and epithelial cells (bladder, lung, oral mucosa).

4. The answer is E. (Reference: p. 425)

The use of genetic testing for evaluation of disease risk, diagnosis, and prognosis will be incorporated into many parts of our lives. It is important to note that the prevalence of genetic disease is not increasing, in contrast to those diseases caused by infectious agents, so that genetic testing should have no negative economic impact on society. In fact, there might be a reduction in the cost of health care and a positive influence on the work force if preventable genetic diseases are appropriately addressed. The prevention of discriminatory practices, education, dissemination of information, and the best uses of such testing are still evolving.

CHAPTER 30 ANSWERS

1. The answer is E. (Reference: p. 430)

In 1991, OSHA published a new occupational health standard designed to prevent exposure to HBV, HIV, and other infectious agents transmitted by contact with blood and other body fluids (29 CFR 1910.1030). The Blood-Borne Pathogens Standard requires that employees with occupational exposure to blood, or other potentially infectious materials (OPIM), be protected through a variety of measures as specified in a written exposure control plan.

2. The answer is D. (Reference: p. 437)

Manual lifting tasks are responsible for a high frequency of acute and chronic back pain complaints among medical center workers, especially among nurses aides, nurses, orderlies, custodians, and laundry and maintenance workers. Studies have consistently shown that nurses aides rank in the top ten occupations at risk for back injury as measured by the number of workers' compensation claims filled per worker (Klein et al., 1984).

3. The answer is C. (Reference: p. 429)

In addition to inspecting patient care areas for hazards particular to patient care providers, non–patient care areas, such as administration, the machine shop, the power plant, and kitchen facilities, should also be inspected carefully. Environmental or area monitoring, as well as personal or breathing zone monitoring for airborne contaminants, should be performed where appropriate as part of the medical center's ongoing hazard assessment program.

4. The answer is A. (Reference: p. 431)

Health care workers employed in urban medical centers that care for large numbers of TB patients are at risk of acquiring occupational TB infection. Every medical center should develop a TB exposure control plan based on traditional principles of TB control (CDC, 1990).

5. The answer is D. (Reference: pp. 436, 437)

The availability and use of Personal Protective Equipment (PPE) are essential to an effective laboratory safety program. Laboratory coats, eye and face protection, and respiratory protection should be used when appropriate. Emergency shower and eyewash facilities should be located in close proximity to areas in the laboratory in which corrosive or irritating chemicals are used.

Section 4

31

Reproductive Hazards

OBJECTIVES

- List pathophysiologic mechanisms of interference with the reproductive process
- Explain what resources are available in order to obtain information regarding adverse reproductive effects
- List guidelines for continuation of work during pregnancy

OUTLINE

VIII. Appendix to Chapter 31: Agents Associated with Adverse Female
       Reproductive Capacity

KEY POINTS

- Concerns about reproductive health are not limited to the pregnant employee in the workplace. While adverse reproductive outcomes may occur as a result of exposure of the fetus in utero, they may also result from toxic exposures experienced by either the male or the female parent before conception occurs. Consequently, concern about the effects of exposures at the workplace on reproductive health is appropriate for pregnant women, for women of childbearing age, and for men.
- In 1991, the Supreme Court prohibited employers from restricting pregnant or fertile women from working in jobs that might injure a fetus and cause an adverse reproductive outcome. Instead, the Court placed the responsibility on the pregnant employee to decide whether to perform duties that might be potentially hazardous to the fetus. The Court placed the responsibility on the company to inform the employee adequately about potential health risks of the work activities.
- In the male, interference with the reproductive process may occur during sperm production. In the female, interference may occur during the production or release of ova, the passage of a fertilized egg through the fallopian tube, or the implantation in the uterus. The embryo may be adversely affected during tissue differentiation or organogenesis. The fetus may not grow normally, resulting in malformations, spontaneous abortions, stillbirths, or premature births. In childhood, subtle developmental effects may become apparent, sometimes years after birth.
- An agent or factor that causes physical birth defects or malformation of the embryo without producing toxicity in the mother is termed a teratogen.
- Principles of teratology include the following: an embryo's susceptibility to teratogenesis depends on its genotype and on its stage of development; teratogens act on developing cells, causing abnormal embryogenesis; the outcomes of teratogenesis may be malformation, growth retardation, functional disorder, or death; the access of teratogenic agents to the target fetal tissues depends on the nature of the teratogenic agents, and the amount of teratogenic effect is related to the dose of the teratogen.
- There is a high background rate of adverse reproductive outcomes in humans. About 10% to 20% of normal conceptions result in spontaneous abortions or stillbirths. Birth defects are recognized in some 3% of live births, of which some two-thirds have no known cause. Only 3% of birth defects have been associated with chemicals or drugs.
- In exploring the medical literature for guidance on a reproductive outcome question, the following are major points to consider: exposure levels, selection of controls, background incidence of events, reliability of ascertainment, multiple exposures, and the interpretation of the findings.
- Animal data can suggest possible human effects, although extrapolation to human experience is problematic.
- Lists of chemicals associated with various adverse reproductive health effects may be found in the medical literature. Additionally, guidelines such as those from the AMA Council of Scientific Affairs are available to assist the physician to determine the length of time into a pregnancy that an employee may continue to work performing various activities.

QUESTIONS

1. A 1991 Supreme Court decision (International Union v. Johnson Controls):

A. requires companies to restrict pregnant women from working in jobs that may injure a fetus.
B. requires companies to restrict women of reproductive age from working in jobs that may injure a fetus.

C. forbids any suit by a child that alleges that the child has been injured in utero by exposure of the mother to reproductive toxins in the workplace.
D. places the responsibility on the employee to decide whether to work in a job that may injure a fetus.
E. protects the employer from being cited under the general duty clause of the Occupational Safety and Health Act of 1970.

2. *Which of the following statements about human reproduction is correct?*

A. The presence in the *male*'s blood of the two *female* reproductive hormones FSH and LH (follicle stimulating hormone and luteinizing hormone) strongly suggests an inborn error of hormone metabolism.
B. The presence of 50 to 150 million sperm per milliliter of ejaculate is an indicator of male infertility.
C. Spermatogenesis in the human male takes 70 to 80 days, or between 2 and 3 months.
D. The human female releases about 50 mature ova during the course of a lifetime of ovulation.
E. Fertilization occurs after implantation of the ovum into the wall of the uterus and is facilitated by conditions that allow the sperm to penetrate the endometrium.

3. *Which of the following statements about human reproduction is **false?***

A. Estrogen deficiency can interfere with the release of ova from the ovary.
B. A delayed or abnormal menstrual period can actually be an early spontaneous abortion.
C. In the human embryo, tissues differentiate into organs (embryonic organogenesis) between the third and the eighth week of gestation.
D. Exposure to ionizing radiation can cause pregnant women to miscarry, but has no effect on the reproductive process in men.
E. The effects of fetotoxins may not become apparent until years after birth.

4. *Which of the following statements regarding human birth defects is true?*

A. The fetus may be more or less susceptible to a teratogen depending on its gestational age.
B. Teratogens usually adversely affect all the cells and tissues of the fetus.
C. Most teratogens cause symptoms in the mother at lower doses than the teratogenic dose.
D. If a pregnant woman is exposed to a teratogen, the fetus always suffers injury.
E. Growth retardation is not a teratogenic effect.

5. *Each of the following variables is known to be associated with adverse human reproductive outcome **except:***

A. the illnesses the father had in childhood.
B. the mother's diet.
C. the mother's smoking history.
D. the father's ethnic background.
E. the recent appendectomy in mother.

6. *With regard to predicting human reproductive effects from animal studies, which of the following statements is true?*

A. The fact that experimental animals and humans may metabolize the chemical differently is irrelevant since the concern is reproductive outcome from exposure to the chemical, not to its metabolites.

B. Since the concentration of the chemical in feed or water is precisely controlled in an animal study, the actual dose ingested is also precisely known.

C. In designing a study of reproductive toxicity, the goal is to look at fetal effects at a precise level of maternal toxicity, measured at between 70% and 85% of the expected normal weight gain during pregnancy for the species.

D. In a well-designed animal study, any adverse effect on the fetus that reaches statistical significance is also necessarily biologically significant.

E. Most compounds that produce reproductive toxicity do so at doses that are close to the dose that produces toxicity in nonpregnant adults of the species.

7. *Which of the following statements regarding usual relative efficiency of routes of administration is **false**?*

A. Ingestion is more efficient than dermal.

B. Dermal is more efficient than inhalation.

C. Intravenous is more efficient than inhalation.

D. Efficiency of various routes of administration of a chemical can be compared by comparing the LD_{50} (the dose that is lethal to 50% of the animals) for the chemical at each route of administration.

E. In the occupational setting, inhalation is a frequent route of exposure.

8. *According to the guidelines from the AMA Council of Scientific Affairs, which of the following regarding human pregnancy and work is true?*

A. North American women who work outside the home are likely to have higher exposures to chemicals at work than at home or in the beauty parlor.

B. A woman experiencing a normal uncomplicated pregnancy should be restricted from secretarial work 4 to 6 weeks prior to the estimated date of delivery.

C. At 3 months of gestation a woman experiencing a normal uncomplicated pregnancy would routinely be restricted from standing more than 4 hours.

D. A woman may climb stairs up to three times per 8-hour shift in the last month of pregnancy.

E. During the first trimester a woman experiencing a normal uncomplicated pregnancy would routinely be restricted from intermittent lifting of more than 50 lb.

REFERENCES

American Medical Association Council on Scientific Affairs. Effects of toxic chemicals on the reproductive system. *J.A.M.A.* 253:3431, 1985.

Bond MB. Role of corporate policy in the control of reproductive hazards of the workplace. *J. Occup. Med.* 28:193, 1986.

International Union v. Johnson Controls, 111 US 1196 (1991).

Logan DC. Reproduction and the workplace: an industry perspective. In: Stein AA, Hatch MC, eds. *Reproductive problems in the workplace. Occupational medicine state of the art review.* Philadelphia: Hanley & Belfus, 1986:473–481.

McLeod J, Ving W. Male fertility potential in terms of semen quality. A review of the past, a study of the present. *Fertil. Steril.* 31:103, 1979.

O'Flaherty, EJ. Absorption, distribution, and elimination of toxic agents. In: Williams PL, Burson JL, eds. *Industrial toxicology, safety and health application in the workplace.* New York: Van Nostrand Reinhold, 1985:47–48.

Radike M. Reproductive toxicology. In: Williams PL, Burson JL, eds. *Industrial toxicology, safety and health applications in the workplace.* New York: Van Nostrand Reinhold, 1985:345.

32

Health Promotion

OBJECTIVES

- List benefits of health promotion programs to the employer
- Explain types of programs that may be included
- Identify methods used to determine the effectiveness of such programs

OUTLINE

    I. Rationale and Justification for Work-Site Health Promotion
        A. Health Care Costs
        B. Absenteeism
        C. Health Risks
        D. Attitudes Toward Health and the Company
   II. Strategic Planning Process
        A. Establishing the Vision, Mission, and Goals
        B. Data Collection
  III. Scope of Programs for Health Promotion
        A. Screening Examinations
        B. Smoking Cessation
        C. Fitness/Aerobics
        D. Nutrition/Cholesterol/Weight Management
        E. Blood Pressure
        F. Stress Management
        G. Employee Assistance Programs
   IV. Implementation Options: What Works and What Doesn't
        A. Who
        B. When
        C. Where
        D. How
    V. Evaluating the Effectiveness of Health Promotion
        A. General Characteristics
        B. Specific Program Evaluation Considerations

    VI. Challenges and Opportunities
   VII. References

KEY POINTS

- Workplace health promotion programs are recognized as an important part of the practice of occupational medicine. Health promotion is the science and art of helping people change their lifestyles through a combination of efforts to enhance awareness, encourage behavior change, and create environments that support good health practices. Such programs have the potential to help control health care costs, impact the utilization of health care, decrease absenteeism, reduce health risks, and improve attitudes.
- Planning is the key to immediate and ongoing success and includes establishing vision, mission, and goals; assessing data; choosing interventions; and determining how results will be measured.
- A variety of health promotion programs may be offered. These include, but are not limited to, screening examinations, smoking cessation programs, fitness/aerobics activities, nutritional or weight management programs, blood pressure screening or monitoring activities, stress management, and employee assistance programs
- Success at the level of participation is the key ingredient to achieving desired program outcomes over time.
- The effectiveness of health promotion activities can be evaluated by the use of process evaluations, measurement of impact, or evaluation of outcomes. The evaluation plan should reflect a consensus, with stated goals that satisfy the interest of all concerned parties.
- A major caution of designing outcome evaluation is that beneficial effects may take years to produce favorable results.

QUESTIONS

*1. Which of the following statements is **not** a valid business reason for establishing a work-site health promotion program?*

A. A health promotion program can foster the well-being of employees.
B. A health promotion program can help control the cost to the company of employees' health care.
C. Health promotion programs help control absenteeism.
D. Companies with more than 50 employees must comply with the federal mandate to establish a health promotion program.
E. Employees' attitudes toward the employer may improve when a company establishes a health promotion program.

2. A modern comprehensive workplace health promotion program will have which of the following characteristics?

A. It will narrowly target one or two easily measurable outcomes.
B. A substantial proportion of its activities will be directed to establishing a work environment that is generally supportive of healthy behavior.
C. Its primary focus will be on encouraging motivated individuals to maintain their fitness.
D. Rather than disciplining employees for using company time to participate in wellness activities, company management will treat grassroots efforts to promote wellness with "benign neglect."
E. Wellness programs for executives will take priority, on the basis that a healthy management is likely to encourage a healthy work environment.

3. *With regard to designing a work-site health promotion program, all of the following contribute to its effectiveness* **except:**

A. identifying the diseases common in the employee population.
B. providing management with a prepackaged lecture program that reviews all major health risks found in the general population.
C. understanding the social makeup of the employee population, including awareness of the ethnic groups, social class, and cultural backgrounds of the employees.
D. having the employees complete baseline and interval health risk appraisals.
E. interviewing management regarding their concerns about employee health behaviors.

4. *All of the following are common elements of work-site health promotion programs* **except:**

A. cholesterol assessment.
B. smoking cessation programs.
C. treatment for drug abuse.
D. blood pressure screening.
E. stress management classes.

5. *Which of the following statements regarding evaluating the effectiveness of work-site health promotion programs is* **false?**

A. Appropriate elements for evaluation include the participants' perceptions of the program, actual changes in their risk factors, and changes in the health status of the employee population as a whole.
B. The time to design a program evaluation is after it has been in place for a year, because it takes at least a year for changes in employees' behavior to become evident and thus amenable to measurement.
C. Typically it is easier to measure the effectiveness of a smoking cessation intervention than a diet modification intervention.
D. The impact of an employee assistance program may be evaluated by looking for changes in liver function tests, changes in patterns of health care utilization, and changes in employee absenteeism.
E. Although stress management courses are difficult to evaluate, it is possible at least to document changes in participants' use of learned coping strategies.

33

The Case Report: Discovery of Occupational Disease

OBJECTIVES

- Explain clinical tools used to identify occupational illness
- Describe the types of clinical observations that are appropriately published in a case report
- Describe how to prepare a case report of a new or unexpected disease association with a particular work setting

OUTLINE

VI. Further Information: Specific Case Reports

KEY POINTS

- To prevent occupational illness, it is first necessary to identify the cause. Case reports of clusters of tumors of unusual type or at unusual anatomic sites have led to the identification of occupational carcinogens.
- The following three elements contribute to a valid and useful case report: an accurate diagnosis, a meticulous exposure history, and a literature review that supports the plausibility of a casual relationship. Likely alternative causes must be excluded.
- The occupational history should be sufficiently detailed to identify the type, intensity, and duration of exposure to materials.
- Some medical conditions may be more likely to be related to workplace factors. A sentinel health event (SHE) is a condition already known to have occupational causes that contributes to unnecessary disease, disability, or untimely death.
- A review of current information in the literature concerning exposure may assist in the determination of causality.
- Characteristics of exposure, such as intensity, duration, and route, and personal characteristics, such as cigarette smoking, alcohol consumption, age, genetic susceptibility, intercurrent disease, and coexposures may interact to influence the ultimate effect on health.
- Exposures may not always be safe simply because levels of exposure are below recommended standards.
- Work practices or personal habits may modify apparently harmless industrial processes.
- Exposures during hobby or home activity may be related to a condition that appears to be due to workplace exposure.
- The diagnosis of occupational illness is often one of exclusion.
- Useful types of case reports include a new disease or condition, a new association between disease and stressor, and an expected development in a disease associated with an exposure, unusual circumstance of exposure, or new data to clarify pathophysiology.
- A typical format for case presentation is as follows: introduction, description of case, other considerations, discussion.

QUESTIONS

1. *You have diagnosed an illness in a patient. In assessing the possible work relatedness of the patient's illness, which of the following items of information is* **least** *helpful?*

A. Temporal relationship of symptoms with exposure at work
B. Family history
C. Company industrial hygiene data regarding levels of exposure
D. Patient's report of co-workers with similar illness
E. Patient's report of hobbies and other nonwork activities

2. *Which of the following circumstances would lead you to investigate further the possibility that a disease is occupational in origin?*

A. You have examined all 22 of the patient's co-workers. None of the others has the disease.
B. A review of the medical literature turns up no previous association between the disease and the patient's type of work.
C. A review of the medical literature turns up no previous association between the disease and the patient's hobbies.

D. The patient's description of working conditions leads you to suspect that exposure control practices at the work site may be less than optimal.

E. The company's safety department supplies you with industrial hygiene monitoring results. These results are the personal monitoring of your patient's co-worker, and they reveal a low level of potential exposure.

3. *Your patient asks you whether it is possible that exposure to a specific chemical at work has caused his/her illness. Which of the following resources is likely to provide helpful information about known toxic effects of the chemical?*

A. The Material Safety Data Sheet (MSDS)

B. A regional office of the National Institute for Occupational Safety and Health (NIOSH)

C. The manufacturer of the chemical

D. Computerized databases such as MEDLINE and TOXLINE

E. All of the above

4. *A group of 15 young Hispanic women work with a catalyst dimethylaminopropionitrile in the foam industry. The previous week the company offered a mass vaccination for influenza, and 60% of the employees, including all the employees in this group, were vaccinated. Today one of the employees mentions to her co-worker that she has been having trouble with urination. The co-worker responds that she has noticed the same thing. Word spreads among their friends, and soon four of these young women have arrived in your clinic requesting evaluation. Leading the list of differential diagnoses is:*

A. autonomic neuropathy from toxic exposure.

B. mass hysteria.

C. venereal disease.

D. a manifestation of insensitive labor relations at work.

E. early manifestation of Guillain-Barré from influenza vaccine.

5. *Each of the following circumstances is appropriate to present as an individual case report in the field of occupational medicine* **except:**

A. the disease has never before been reported in association with this type of exposure.

B. a team consisting of a research biochemist, an electrophysiologist, and a neurotoxicologist has identified the biochemical site of action of a newly identified neurotoxin.

C. the index patient is an immigrant and unusual constituents in the patient's diet may have interacted with the workplace chemical exposure to cause the disease.

D. the disease has never before been reported; you believe it is a new disease.

E. while the condition is a common infectious disease, in this patient it followed an unusual pattern of relapse and remission, with each relapse following an exposure to a chemical that was recently introduced to the patient's place of work.

REFERENCES

Kreiss K, et al. Neurological dysfunction of the bladder in workers exposed to dimethylaminopropionitrile. *J.A.M.A.* 243:741, 1980.

Whorton MD, et al. Infertility in male pesticide workers. *Lancet* 2:1259, 1977.

34

Economics of Occupational Medicine

OBJECTIVES

- Explain how occupational health services can support an organization
- List the traditional occupational medical services
- List newer occupational services that may support an organization
- Explain the impact of lifestyle on health and costs
- Describe how occupational health services can be consistent with and support the mission, goals, and objectives of an organization
- List newer occupational services, and describe how they may support an organization
- Describe the impact of lifestyle on health of employees and costs of maintaining their health
- Explain how to evaluate the economic benefits of occupational health services and how to communicate these benefits effectively to management

OUTLINE

   I. Traditional Occupational Medical Services
- A. Preplacement, Disability, and Return-to-Work Examinations
- B. Medical Surveillance
- C. Immunization
- D. Treatment of Job-Related Injuries and Illnesses
- E. Rehabilitation and Return-to-Work
- F. Consulting Activities
- G. Industrial Hygiene Consultation

  II. Newer Occupational Services
- A. Employee Assistance Programs
- B. Work Hardening
- C. On-Site Management of Nonoccupational Illness and Injuries
- D. Chronic Disease Management

KEY POINTS

- The mission, goals, and objectives of an occupational health program should be congruent with and support the mission, goals, and objectives of the organization.
- Economic benefits of both traditional and newer occupational health services can be evaluated and used to justify existing or new programs.
- Adverse health effects from the workplace may be identified by medical surveillance and prevented by control of any hazardous exposures identified by the surveillance exams.
- Traditional occupational medical services may include preplacement, disability, and return-to-work examinations, medical surveillance activities, immunizations, and the treatment of job-related injuries and illnesses. In addition to providing treatment, the occupational medicine physician acts as the medical liaison with the private medical community. Other activities may include rehabilitation services, consulting activities, and industrial hygiene consultation.
- The traditional cornerstone of clinical occupational health programs is the determination of the ability of an applicant or employee to perform work. The Americans with Disabilities Act (ADA) has sharpened the focus of this activity, since it requires the employer to make a thorough attempt to reasonably accommodate an applicant or employee if such accommodation will allow the individual to perform the essential functions of the job. A beneficial side effect of making such accommodations is that making changes in the way work is performed may actually make jobs safer for all employees. Consequently, when evaluating the economic costs of performing the medical screening and placement programs, it is appropriate to balance against those costs the savings incurred by preventing work-related injuries.
- A key duty of the occupational health professional is to monitor health-related data on members of the work force exposed to chemical, radiation, and other physical hazards and to compare the values for exposed and unexposed groups periodically. Where significant differences are noted, and where assessment of the employees and the work site leads to the conclusion that the discrepancies are work-related, the exposure should be quantified and controlled.

- Immunization can be instituted to prevent occupational transmission of infectious disease, as in hepatitis B immunization of workers in health care facilities, prisons, and sanitation industries. It can also be instituted as a cost-containment measure, as in the case of immunization of workers against tetanus, thus preventing many visits to medical facilities for prophylaxis of minor wounds.
- Treatment of injuries and illnesses on site can be cost effective. Time lost in travel off-site and waiting for treatment is avoided, and the actual cost of treatment is often less. Also, physicians and nurses who are familiar with the work environment may be more efficient in addressing issues around recovery. Where on-site care is not possible, community-based occupational health services can also save time by prompt treatment and effective management of work-related injuries.
- Knowledge of the job is critical for appropriate placement of workers returning to work following an illness or injury. Early return to work benefits both the employee and the employer.
- Occupational medicine professionals often serve as internal consultants to an organization in areas of industrial hygiene, job modification, employee assistance, and other special problems. These activities are directed toward prevention of health problems. In particular, occupational health practitioners may prevent illnesses and injuries caused by chemical and physical hazards at the work site by advising managers about the presence, nature, and magnitude of hazards. They can also evaluate the effectiveness of protection against the hazards, both by on-site inspection and by epidemiologic surveillance. These activities are best conducted in close cooperation with the industrial hygienist.
- Newer occupational medical services include employee assistance programs, work hardening, on-site management of non–work-related health problems, assistance with the management of chronic disease, self-care instruction and counseling, and case management services. In addition, work-site health promotion programs are increasingly common.
- At most work sites, a small proportion of employees are responsible for a large proportion of the absentee days. Many of these employees suffer from somatization of psychological conflicts. Employee assistance programs (EAPs) can assist with resolution of these conflicts with cost-benefit ratios of up to 10:1.
- Injury and reinjury in taxing jobs can be prevented by gradually increasing work load.
- Many employers, especially those who are self-insured, have noted the advantages of providing comprehensive health care for both occupational and nonoccupational illnesses and injuries at the work site. Employees receive earlier treatment with reduced morbidity, better health supervision, ready access to practitioners who understand the work environment, and lower unit cost. Occupational health programs designed to serve smaller companies in the immediate geographic area can have similar benefits to an organization.
- Management of such conditions as hypercholesterolemia, diabetes, and hypertension may be more effective at the work site, primarily because of ease of access to medical care, close follow-up, and coordination with managing physicians.
- Education of patients in self-care for minor illnesses and injuries has reduced health care costs. Furthermore, educating employees in the best way to use the medical care system has resulted in increases in the quality of care and decreases in inappropriate utilization.
- Close management of seriously ill, injured, or chronically ill employees or those undergoing treatment helps to avoid unnecessary procedures, to ensure appropriate therapy, and to coordinate proper discharge planning and early return to work.
- Health promotion at the work site has flourished since the recognition that costs for lifestyle-related problems are some 10 to 15 times greater than costs for work-related illnesses and injuries.

- There is evidence from both epidemiologic studies and clinical trials to show that morbidity and mortality are reduced if risk factors are decreased.
- Early detection of hypertension, hypercholesterolemia, and cervical and breast cancer has a significant benefit-cost ratio. Many other common screening tests, when conducted in asymptomatic individuals, are of minimal value and may result in additional costs to rule out false positives.
- Medical benefits quality and cost management are relatively new to many occupational medicine physicians. Their advice can be of great value to a company's benefits organization by recommending appropriate medical services to be covered, including preventive services and by supporting reimbursement schemes that discourage the use of medically unnecessary services.
- Occupational medicine physicians can assist benefits managers in selecting among various approaches to utilization management, such as use of a gatekeeper to authorize hospitalizations and certain procedures, redesign of benefits plans to discourage inappropriate utilization, and capitated payment systems to health care providers.

QUESTIONS

1. The goals and objectives of an occupational health program should be consistent with:

A. ethical professional conduct.
B. cost-effective, value-added care.
C. the mission, goals, and objectives of the client or sponsoring employers.
D. prevention of adverse health effects from the workplace.
E. all of the above.

*2. The role of the occupational health professional should include all **except:***

A. liaisons with the nonoccupational medical community.
B. evaluators of care financed by medical benefits programs.
C. health promotion.
D. protection of employees from occupational hazards.
E. discussion of confidential medical information with corporate executives.

3. Cost-effective screening for cumulative trauma disorders (CTDs) can be accomplished by:

A. regular inquiries of workers about discomfort in the wrists, arms, shoulders, and back.
B. oblique views of the lumbar spine.
C. periodic testing of nerve conduction velocities of median nerves.
D. annual physicals.
E. all of the above.

4. Which of the following observations regarding medical surveillance is true?

A. When calculating the benefits of medical surveillance, only the actual medical costs of the prevented injuries or illnesses should be included.
B. The occupational physician should be involved in analysis of group health data from the employee population only if the organization does not have an epidemiologist to perform this activity.
C. In general, the costs of preventing occupational illnesses or injuries through engineering controls outweigh the medical costs of treating the conditions.

D. The economic value of medical surveillance and resulting preventive activities can be calculated if the probability of illness is known for the levels of exposure present in the facility.
E. There is no need for ongoing surveillance of a population exposed to hazards whose health effects are already known.

5. *Immunizations are least necessary for the prevention of occupational illness in which of the following occupations?*

A. Prison guard
B. Sanitation worker
C. Hospital janitor
D. Project engineer
E. Day care worker

6. *Regarding an employee's return to work after an absence due to illness, the following statements are all true* **except:**

A. EAPs can prevent hospitalization of employees with mental health problems by directing them to outpatient treatment that emphasizes early rehabilitation.
B. Placing an employee in a work-hardening program that gradually increases the work load may prevent reinjury by allowing acclimation over time.
C. When an employee has a performance problem, there is always a mental health component; consequently the EAP should provide medical or counseling referrals to all such employees.
D. The occupational physician often benefits the local medical community by establishing predictable and appropriate referral patterns.
E. When a patient returns to work from a nonoccupational illness, the occupational physician is in a position to recommend modified work duties that will be appropriate to the work setting and to the employee.

REFERENCES

Bureau of National Affairs. *Alcohol and drugs in the workplace: costs, controls, and controversies.* Washington, DC: Bureau of National Affairs, 1986.
Recommendation of the Immunization Practice Advisory Committee. Prevention and control of influenza. *M.M.W.R.* 34:261, 1985.
Recommendations for protection against viral hepatitis. *M.M.W.R.* 34:23, 1985.

35

Educational Opportunities

OBJECTIVES

- Describe the role of occupational medicine in the provision of medical care in the United States
- Describe the components of residency training programs in occupational medicine
- List available training programs that help primary care physicians improve their knowledge about occupational and environmental medicine
- Describe other information resources in occupational and environmental medicine

OUTLINE

KEY POINTS

- There is an estimated shortage of 3,100 to 5,500 physicians with special competence in occupational and environmental medicine.
- The Institute of Medicine (IOM) has recommended that all primary care physicians should be able to identify possible occupationally or environmentally induced conditions and make appropriate referrals for follow-up.

- Occupational and environmental medicine is a specialty that focuses on the prevention of illness and injury at work.
- The Residency Review Committee (RRC) of the Accreditation Council for Graduate Medical Education (ACGME) provides oversight and accreditation for occupational medicine residency training programs.
- The American Board of Preventive Medicine (ABPM) administers board certification in occupational medicine. Pathways for eligibility to sit for the certifying examination include completion of an accredited residency in occupational medicine followed by a period of relevant practice experience or an alternative pathway that requires, in addition to specific medical training, successful completion of graduate-level courses in biostatistics, epidemiology, health services administration, and environmental health. Requirements for board certification are periodically revised.
- NIOSH has established Educational Resource Centers (ERCs) to provide multidisciplinary educational resources in occupational health. These centers provide continuing medical education (CME) opportunities. They have also created a comprehensive curriculum for use by primary care residency training programs to teach the fundamentals of occupational and environmental medicine to nonspecialists.
- The American College of Occupational and Environmental Medicine (ACOEM) sponsors seminars and courses related to the specialty. These programs are offered each spring and fall in conjunction with national meetings.

QUESTIONS

1. *The IOM has recommended that "all primary care physicians be able to identify possible occupationally or environmentally induced conditions and make appropriate referrals for follow-up." Of the following, what is the **least** useful CME topic to help meet this goal?*

A. Review of epidemiology of hepatitis B
B. Review of epidemiology of disease in the vicinity of Superfund sites
C. Update in suturing techniques for lacerations
D. Overview of federal regulations on blood-borne pathogens
E. Review of criteria used by state workers' compensation commissions to determine whether to require second opinions prior to surgery

2. *The Accreditation Council for Graduate Medical Education (ACGME) requires some element of occupational medical training in which of the following residencies?*

A. Orthopedic surgery
B. Family practice
C. Dermatology
D. Obstetrics
E. None of the above

3. *Which of the following statements regarding the specialty of occupational and environmental medicine is **false**?*

A. It is a specialty that focuses on disease prevention.
B. A major element of data collection in this specialty is observing employees at the work site.
C. Much of the disease prevention in this specialty occurs as a result of the physician providing advice to company management.
D. Typically, the majority of an occupational physician's patient population is healthy.

E. The possession of excellent clinical skills is all a physician needs to deliver competent occupational medical services.

4. *Major sources of funding for occupational medicine residency training include all the following* **except:**

A. hospitals, in exchange for inpatient services.
B. a scholarship fund established by the ACOEM.
C. the National Institute of Occupational Safety and Health (NIOSH).
D. financial grants from corporations.
E. income from consultative services provided by the occupational medicine program.

5. *Which of the following statements regarding residency training of occupational and environmental medicine physicians is true?*

A. While there is a slight excess of residency-trained occupational medicine physicians in the United States, this is being addressed by reducing the number of occupational medicine programs.
B. Because the ACGME provides oversight and accreditation for in-hospital residency programs only, it does not provide accreditation for occupational and environmental residency programs.
C. Nationwide, occupational and environmental residency programs graduate some 75 to 100 physicians annually.
D. Occupational and environmental medicine residency programs consist entirely of classroom didactic study of such subjects as epidemiology, biostatistics, and health services administration.
E. Occupational and environmental medicine residency programs consist of 3 years of clinical work, which is divided approximately evenly among large corporation medical departments, hospital occupational health departments, state health departments, and free-standing occupational health clinics.

6. *A physician trained in another specialty may wish to learn more about occupational and environmental medicine without going through an entire residency program. Which of the following statements regarding potential sources of information is true?*

A. NIOSH-funded ERCs provide training programs that are designed specifically for safety professionals and industrial hygienists; thus, only rarely do they contain information that is useful for physicians.
B. While schools of public health offer courses in biostatistics and epidemiology, these focus on general topics, such as the control of infectious disease, and offer little insight into occupational and environmental medicine issues.
C. The postgraduate courses offered by the ACOEM are open only to member physicians.
D. One objective of ACOEM's basic curriculum is to provide nonoccupational medicine specialists with a useful overview of occupational medicine topics.
E. Occupational medicine is too small a specialty to provide much active participation in state medical societies.

REFERENCES

American Medical Association. *Directory of graduate medical education programs.* Chicago: AMA, 1992.
Institute of Medicine. *Role of the primary care physician in occupational and environmental medicine.* Washington, DC: National Academy Press, 1988.

36

Computers in Occupational Medical Practice

OBJECTIVES

- Explain how computers may benefit the practice of occupational medicine
- Describe guidelines for evaluation and selection of computer software
- Describe components of an occupational medicine information system

OUTLINE

KEY POINTS

- Computers are used in occupational medical practice to automate office processes and for a variety of medical applications. Some uses include the generation of random numbers or the preparation of reports mandated by regulatory agencies.
- Computerization allows improved efficiency and productivity, enhanced quality, decision making, and regulatory compliance.
- Occupational health information systems have paralleled the evolution of computer systems, ranging from first-generation mainframe programs and minicomputer systems to the modern personal computers (PCS), with linkage to modems, scanners, and medical testing equipment. The ability to network with personal computers allows multiple users and raises significant questions about confidentiality of medical records.
- Contemporary case management systems contribute to quality improvement and cost-containment initiatives.
- Computerized case management systems can feature disability duration guidelines, medical protocols, and sophisticated scheduling and follow-up programs.
- Implementation of integrated health data management systems can help to prevent unnecessary duplication of effort, foster coordination among units, and provide a clearer picture of a company's health expenditures and priorities.
- Some components of an occupational health information system may include automation of office work, maintenance of updated personnel information, benefits information, work history and job tracking, functional requirements of jobs, work restrictions, appointment scheduling, regulatory requirements, medical record keeping, health history, medical examination results, medical treatment, injury management, case management, health promotion, drug and alcohol testing, employee assistance programs (EAPs), medical surveillance, exposure monitoring, chemical inventory, toxicology data, safety programs, financial information, and epidemiologic efforts.
- Occupational health information systems of the future will be based on the personal computers that are networked and are expected to use a graphics user interface with advanced software systems. Testing equipment will be connected to the system, and there will be connections to other company applications (or departments), allowing increased production and flexibility.

QUESTIONS

1. *Which of the following computer-based capabilities is least likely to be of much use in an occupational medical practice?*

A. A random number generator
B. Word processing software
C. Forms for injury reporting
D. Computer assisted design (CAD) software
E. Electronic mail

2. *Benefits of an automated occupational medicine clinic management system include all **except** which one of the following?*

A. Increased efficiency, productivity, and accuracy
B. Enhanced quality and decision making
C. Reduced office personnel costs
D. Regulatory compliance and litigation assistance
E. Provision of additional supplemental services

3. *The application of computers that contributes most to their successful integration into an occupational medicine practice is support of the office staff in the pursuit of everyday tasks. To serve this purpose, which of the following would be most valuable?*

A. Interactive medical histories
B. Injury reporting
C. Clinical decision support/practice guidelines
D. Telecommunications access to databases
E. General office automation

4. *Integrated Health Data Management Systems (IHDMSs) and Occupational Health Information Systems (OHISs) can potentially have a bewildering variety of components. Possible users of the system include medical, human resources, safety, and industrial hygiene. Each of these possible users could reasonably and ethically have access to all of the following elements **except:***

A. word processing.
B. an employee's demographic data (name, mailing address, social security number).
C. an individual employee's job capabilities and work restrictions.
D. EAP records.
E. a chemical inventory.

37

Training and Communications

OBJECTIVES

- Explain general types of training mandated by government agencies
- Describe the hazard communication standard
- Explain information included in the Material Safety Data Sheet (MSDS)

OUTLINE

KEY POINTS

- Many standards promulgated by the Occupational Safety and Health Administration (OSHA) explicitly require the employer to train employees in the safety and health aspects of their jobs or make it the employer's responsibility to limit certain job assignments to employees who are certified, competent, or qualified.

- An effective program of safety and health training for workers can result in fewer accidents and illnesses, better morale, and lower insurance premiums, among other benefits.
- Training requirements of OSHA are found in the Code of Federal Regulations (CFR).
- At virtually any manufacturing facility that employs ten workers or more, some fundamental training requirements are mandatory: fire protection, respirator use, hearing conservation, process safety management, and medical services.
- OSHA requires each employer to develop detailed emergency plans and fire prevention plans.
- Other regulations include requirements for eye and face protection, respiratory protection, occupational head protection, occupational foot protection, and electrical protective devices. Employers are required to arrange medical certification for workers who need respirators in the course of their work. It is up to the judgment of the examining physician as to whether a person can be medically cleared for respirator use.
- Employees who are exposed to noise at or above an 8-hour time-weighted average (TWA) of 85 dB must be enrolled in a yearly training program instituted by their employer.
- The Emergency Planning and Community Right-to-Know Act of 1986, known as Title III of the Superfund Amendments and Reauthorization Act (SARA), mandates that every facility using, storing, or manufacturing hazardous chemicals make public its inventory and report every release of a hazardous chemical to public officials and health personnel. Every facility must also cooperate with physicians who are treating victims of hazardous chemical exposure.
- OSHA has issued a Process Safety Management of Highly Hazardous Chemicals regulation that requires every employee involved in operating processes to receive initial and refresher training on specific safety and health hazards emergency operations.

QUESTIONS

1. Which of the following statements regarding standards promulgated by the OSHA is true?

A. OSHA standards are related to safety, such as fire protection, contractor safety, and equipment standards, and do not address medical issues or involve occupational physicians.

B. At almost any manufacturing facility where ten or more workers are employed, OSHA requires some employee training.

C. Since OSHA-mandated safety training falls under the purview of the safety department, tact dictates that the occupational physician refrain from questioning employees regarding their understanding of safety practices.

D. OSHA requires employers of ten workers or more to maintain a medical emergency response team that is trained in cardiopulmonary resuscitation.

E. Under OSHA standards, prior to implementation of the emergency action plan, the employer is required to review the plan only with those who are members of emergency response teams.

2. With reference to OSHA's standards specifically addressing personal protective equipment (CFR 1910.132- CFR 1910.140), which of the following statements is true?

A. Employers may avoid the requirement to train workers about the hazardous aspects of their jobs by instead training them in the proper use of personal protective equipment.

B. Unless an employer has an unusually thin face, a beard, or an active case of severe acne, any NIOSH-certified respirator will provide an adequate seal.

C. If an individual has a beard, it is acceptable to use petrolatum jelly along the edge of the respirator to increase air tightness.
D. If an employee has a forced respirator volume in 1 second (FEV₁) of less than 70% predicted, OSHA requires physicians to restrict the individual from respirator use in any but emergency situations.
E. OSHA has not established spirometry criteria that an employee must pass in order for the physician to clear the employee to wear a respirator.

3. *Which of the following is a required element of the OSHA-mandated training program for hearing conservation?*

A. Employees who are exposed to noise at or above 85 dB 8-hour TWA must be trained.
B. The training program must be annual.
C. The training program must describe the effects of noise on hearing.
D. The training program must describe hearing tests and explain their purpose.
E. All of the above.

4. *Which of the following statements regarding provision of first-aid and medical services is **false**?*

A. Under OSHA regulations, if community medical care is not readily available, the employer must arrange for individuals trained in first aid to provide care.
B. If strong acids, strong alkalis, or other corrosive chemicals are present in the workplace, OSHA requires that eyewash facilities and showers must be provided in the work area.
C. NIOSH approves first-aid equipment.
D. OSHA leaves to the discretion of the employer exactly what medical and first-aid supplies are to be available at the work site.
E. First-aid supplies appropriate to the facility's processes and history of previous injuries should be readily available.

5. *Which of the following statements regarding the Hazard Communication Standard is true?*

A. It is an EPA standard first promulgated in 1993.
B. It applies only to manufacturers, importers, and distributors of hazardous chemicals.
C. It applies only to companies that handle hazardous chemicals that are in a quantity and form that might endanger the surrounding community.
D. It applies to OSHA-covered employers that handle hazardous chemicals.
E. The standard outlines in detail exactly what steps an employer must take in order to be in compliance.

6. *Which of the following statements about Material Safety Data Sheets (MSDSs) is **false**?*

A. A properly worded MSDS will provide information regarding health effects of the chemical.
B. The MSDS may provide useful information to medical personnel regarding how to treat an overexposure to the chemical.
C. A major purpose of properly worded MSDS is to remove legal responsibility for safe handling of the chemical from the manufacturer and place it on the employee who actually uses the chemical.

D. A MSDS will describe the proper personal protective equipment to use when handling the chemical.
E. If a treating physician or nurse needs to know the specific chemical identity in order to treat a medical emergency, and if that information is not present on the MSDS, the manufacturer is required to inform the physician or nurse immediately of the identity of the chemical.

*7. OSHA's laboratory standard specifically lists all of the following types **except:***

A. carcinogens.
B. hepatitis B.
C. reproductive toxins.
D. irritants.
E. hepatotoxins.

REFERENCES

Garbo MJ, et al. OSHA Hazard Communication Standard, helping prevent chemical hazards. *A.A.O.H.N. J.* 36:366, 1988.
Kilby JA. New OSHA standard goes into effect regarding safety in laboratories. *Occup. Health Saf.* May 1990:82.
O'Neill BM, et al. Right-to-know laws: a guide to maintaining compliance. *Occup. Health Saf.* June 1988:28–49.

38

International Occupational Health

OBJECTIVES

- Describe the importance of international travel on occupational medical practice
- List various components of medical kits for international travelers
- Explain issues important in management of traveler's diarrhea

OUTLINE

KEY POINTS

- The proliferation of international business has led many occupational physicians to become knowledgeable in international affairs and to direct occupational health programs at great distance.
- The occupational physician may have to manage pretravel preparation, assist with strategies to maintain health for the international traveler, and perform routine health screening of employees on their return.
- To ensure good health when overseas, it may be necessary to identify individuals with chronic medical problems and to assure adequate prescriptions for treatment. Medications may be needed for prevention of diseases and other conditions that may develop in transit.
- The traveling employee will need to be current on required vaccines and may wish to take advantage of recommended vaccines.
- Routine screening tests are often recommended for returning travelers to detect acquired diseases. The types of screening tests may vary according to the countries visited and the presence of symptoms.
- Traveler's diarrhea is a pervasive ailment. Prophylaxis and/or treatment of simple traveler's diarrhea can usually be achieved with bismuth-salicylate (Pepto-Bismol), 2 tablets q.i.d. Prophylactic antibiotics may be appropriate for short-term visitors to certain countries.

QUESTIONS

*1. Which of the following services is **least** appropriate to provide employees assigned to work overseas?*

A. Developing protocols to guide overseas employees in treating common medical conditions
B. Performing baseline medical examinations prior to overseas assignments
C. Developing medical guidelines to assist human resources personnel in selection of employees for overseas assignments
D. Orienting employees to medical services that may be encountered overseas
E. Providing prophylactic penicillin by injection prior to travel

*2. Which of the following items should **not** be included in a medical kit for travelers to developing countries?*

A. Pharmaceuticals that are readily available in the destination country's local pharmacies.
B. Prescription medications for the employee's personal medical conditions.
C. Signed prescriptions for medications that are already in the medical kit.
D. A signed statement from the physician that the country's requirements for vaccination are medically unnecessary.
E. A signed statement from the physician listing the medications in the kit and confirming that they are medically necessary for the traveler.

3. *With regard to avoiding water-borne diseases, which of the following statements is **false?***

A. Drinking only carbonated bottled water decreases the likelihood that local tap water has been substituted for the original bottled water.
B. Adding chlorine or iodine to cloudy water and allowing it to sit for a full 10 minutes will eliminate risk from viruses.
C. In modern cities such as Paris or Berlin there is a genuine risk that the tap water may have been contaminated through leakage into ancient water pipes.
D. Heating water to 62°C for a full 10 minutes will eliminate risk of bacterial illness.
E. The addition of iodine to water after filtering with "Katadyn" filter almost completely eliminates risk from viruses.

4. *With regard to reducing or preventing jet lag, which of the following statements is **false?***

A. Eating pasta or other carbohydrate rich foods the night before the trip, then eating light meals of fruit and salads during travel, are recommended dietary approaches to reduce jet lag.
B. Jet lag may be partially prevented by looking out the window of the airplane during a flight to Japan.
C. Alcohol suppresses the rapid eye movement (REM) phase of sleep and should be avoided during the entire trip.
D. Travelers should avoid excessive water or other fluid intake the day prior to travel.
E. At altitude, taking triazolam (Halcion) in conjunction with alcohol may result in retrograde amnesia.

5. *Which of the following observations regarding screening a traveler who has returned from an overseas assignment is **false?***

A. It is reasonable to obtain hepatitis B serology in previously unvaccinated individuals who have spent time in rural China.
B. Examination of the skin for rashes, nodules, or edema is indicated in individuals returning from an extended visit in rural areas of Central or South America.
C. A tuberculin skin test is indicated in individuals returned from visiting refugee camps in Asia.
D. Serologic tests for schistosomiasis or filariasis are still too new and unreliable to perform as a routine screen on asymptomatic individuals who have visited rural areas where those diseases are endemic.
E. A tuberculin skin test is indicated for individuals returned from working in a facility located in rural Italy.

6. *Which of the following statements regarding traveler's diarrhea is **false?***

A. Prophylactic antibiotics are unnecessary for travelers who meticulously follow the CDC recommendations in eating and drinking.
B. Doxycycline 100 mg/d is one recommended regimen for prophylaxis of traveler's diarrhea.
C. Trimethoprim/sulfamethoxazole, one tablet per day, is a recommended regimen for prophylaxis of traveler's diarrhea.
D. Bismuth-salicylate (Pepto-Bismol), 2 tablets q.i.d., is a recommended regimen for prophylaxis of traveler's diarrhea.
E. Prophylactic antibiotics are optional for short-term (less than a week) visitors to Mexico, but are medically necessary when an individual will be spending several months.

7. *With regards to AIDS and HIV, which of the following statements would **not** be appropriate advice to overseas travelers?*

A. If the individual is traveling to some countries in Asia or Africa, it is prudent to carry a report of negative HIV testing that has been signed by the physician, since this may be required by customs.
B. Disposable syringes and needles should be included in the medical kit for travelers to countries where HIV/AIDS is endemic and medical services are of variable quality.
C. Since the blood supply in some countries may not be free of HIV, travelers are well advised to avoid activities likely to result in injuries that might require blood transfusions.
D. Casual heterosexual activity is not a likely way of contracting AIDS while traveling in Europe.
E. A country's blood supply may be contaminated with HIV because the country lacks the financial resources to test the blood supply or because the country refuses to acknowledge that its citizenry might indulge in practices associated with HIV transmission.

REFERENCES

Gustatsson LL. *Handbook of drugs for tropical parasitic infections.* London: Taylor and Francis, 1987.
Warren KS. *Tropical and geographical medicine.* New York: McGraw-Hill, 1985.
Steffan R, et al. Efficacy and side effects of six agents in the self-treatment of traveler's diarrhea. *Travel Med. Int. J.* 6:153, 1988.

39

Workers' Compensation

OBJECTIVES

- Describe the evolution of workers' compensation in the United States
- Describe trends in the rate of occupational illness and injury
- Explain the types of benefits available from workers' compensation
- Describe incentives and disincentives relating to workers' compensation
- Explain the importance of medical management of injury cases

OUTLINE

IX. Appendix to Chapter 39: BLS Estimates of Occupational Injury and Illness Incidence Rates for Selected Industries, 1989

KEY POINTS

- Prior to the development of workers' compensation in the United States, injured workers had to prove that their injuries were due to employer negligence, which resulted in a slow, costly, and uncertain legal process. As a defense, the employer could claim that the employee contributed to the injury, that he or she had assumed risk by taking the job, or that negligent acts of fellow workers were responsible for the injury.
- Accidental work deaths have declined 81% between 1912 and 1990. The top five occupational causes of deaths are motor vehicle accidents (35.5%), falls (12.7%), electric current accidents (3.6%), burns (3.5%), and noningestive poisonings (3.5%).
- Back injuries have been the largest category of body parts injured for several years, accounting for 22% of cases and 31% of compensation costs.
- Workers' compensation laws represented a compromise or lesser peril for both employers and employees. These laws were supposed to ensure rapid payment to injured workers for lost wages and medical costs regardless of fault. In exchange, employer's liability for occupational injuries, illness, and death was limited.
- All industrial and most service employment is covered by workers' compensation statutes; however, farm labor, domestic service, and casual employees are usually exempted from the laws.
- Merchant marine and railroad workers are generally not covered by state workers' compensation acts, but may seek damage under the Federal Employee Liability Act (FELA).
- Workers' compensation provides benefits for wage replacement, medical and legal expenses, and permanent impairment. Most states limit compensation to two-thirds of previous wages and cover all medical costs.
- Companies generally find it less expensive to purchase workers' compensation insurance than to invest in loss control technology or prevention.
- Company policy may remove incentives for managers to allow limited duty for injured workers. This disincentive clearly prevents rapid return to work, which is associated with shorter recovery times and reduced payments. The availability of light work or modified duties is key to a reduction in accident severity rates.
- Medical management of workers' compensation cases is necessary because of wide variations in the quality and quantity of medical care and the absence of medical expertise under the existing property and casualty insurance framework.

QUESTIONS

*1. Which of the following statements regarding workers' compensation is **false?***

A. A major contributor to the high cost of medical expenses under workers' compensation is the fragmented delivery of medical care.
B. Wage replacement costs under workers' compensation are increasing at almost twice the rate of the general wage index.
C. Medical care costs under workers' compensation are rising two to three times as fast as the medical consumer price index.
D. Attempts to control the medical costs of workers' compensation frequently cause the quality of patient care to deteriorate.
E. Work-related injuries have resulted in an increase in number of lost workdays per 100 employees over the past several years.

2. The most commonly reported part of the body involved in occupational injuries is:

A. the eye.

B. the wrist.
C. the neck.
D. the back.
E. the ankle.

3. *Which of the following statements regarding occupational deaths is **false**?*

A. The most common cause of occupational death is motor vehicle accidents.
B. Explosions are one of the five most common causes of occupational death.
C. Most authorities believe that the number of work-related deaths is understated.
D. More occupational deaths occur from falls than from electric current accidents, burns, and toxic exposures combined.
E. Occupational death rates trended downward in the 1970s and 1980s.

4. *Which of the following statements regarding the scope of workers' compensation laws is true?*

A. All full-time workers in the United States are covered by workers' compensation insurance.
B. Benefits under the Federal Social Security Disability Program are financed by an experience-based tax on employers.
C. Between 75% and 80% of individuals disabled from occupational disease are covered by workers' compensation.
D. Under most state laws, individuals may file for workers' compensation benefits at any time after they develop a compensable disease.
E. Workers' compensation laws are not consistent from state to state.

5. *Which of the following statements regarding the costs of workers' compensation is **false**?*

A. The National Council on Compensation Insurance estimated that in 1991 total workers' compensation expenditures for wage replacement, administrative and legal costs, and medical costs was approximately $60 billion.
B. By 1992, the average cost of the medical portion of a workers' compensation case was over $6,000.
C. Under most state laws, all medical bills for an occupational injury must be paid.
D. Workers' compensation costs average between 3% and 5% of payroll for most employers.
E. In general, Medicare, Medicaid, and private insurance have been more successful in containing the costs of medical care than workers' compensation insurance has been.

6. *Which of the following statements regarding typical workers' compensation benefits required by most states workers' compensation laws is true?*

A. A major reason for employers to self-insure is that they are then required to provide only a portion of the benefits that are provided under state statutes.
B. Under workers' compensation rules, impairment and disability mean substantially the same thing.
C. Benefits include replacement of wages up to a maximum percentage of the worker's preinjury wage.
D. All injured employees receive lump sum awards, either on return to work or on the occasion that they are determined to be permanently unable to return to work.

E.   Payment of an injured employee's medical bills related to the injury is capped at a dollar limit that is specified by state regulation for each category of medical condition.

7. *Disincentives to cost containment in the workers' compensation system include all of the following **except** which one?*

A.   Usually it costs less to pay workers' compensation insurance premiums than to install the engineering controls that would prevent accidents.
B.   Workers' compensation insurance premiums are designed to cover up to 10 years of reimbursement (the "tail") for injuries that occur in a given year; thus, improvements that a company makes would have no significant impact on the cost of workers' compensation insurance for up to 10 years.
C.   Spreading risk across insurance pools or large employee populations reduces the cost to the individual employer of a major accident and, thus, reduces the financial motivation to prevent such an accident.
D.   Many corporations do not charge workers' compensation costs back to the department (or even the facility) where the accident occurred, thus reducing the motivation of local management to prevent accidents.
E.   At most companies an individual employee's health benefits cover more costs and are easier to use than the workers' compensation system, so employees will shift the costs for work-related injuries to their own health insurance.

8. *All of the following statements regarding the workers' compensation system in the United States are true **except** which one?*

A.   Medical services provided under workers' compensation statutes vary widely in quantity and quality.
B.   Workers' compensation claims adjusters often have no medical background.
C.   There are no reliable studies available to assist in predicting the expected length of disability in cases of uncomplicated low back pain.
D.   Workers' compensation cases are often maintained open for years, with no medical evaluation or reassessment that might demonstrate a significant change in the patient's impairment status.
E.   When selecting physicians to serve on preferred provider panels for workers' compensation cases, it is important to consider the physicians' skills in patient interactions in addition to their medical competence.

REFERENCES

Deyo RA, Diehl AK, Rosenthal M. How many days of bed rest for acute low back pain? A randomized clinical trial. *N. Engl. J. Med.* 315:1064, 1986.

Doyle R, et al. *Health care management guidelines, vol 3: ambulatory care guidelines.* Seattle: Milliman and Robertson, 1990.

Harris JS, et al. *Medical disability standards for orthopaedic disorders.* Brentwood, TN: Focus Health Care Management, 1989.

National Council on Compensation Insurance. *Issues report, 1992.* New York: NCCI, 1992.

Reed PR. *The medical disability advisor.* New York: LRP, 1990.

40

Health Care Management

OBJECTIVES

- Describe types of involvement by occupational physicians in workplace health issues
- Explain health care cost containment strategies employed by business
- Describe methods used by occupational physicians to participate in health care management systems

OUTLINE

  I. Health Care Management
    A. Personal Illness
      1. Employer-Based Insurance
        Figure 40–1. Average annual wages versus average annual health plan costs.
        Figure 40–2. Rise in employer spending, 1970 to 1989 per full-time employee.
      2. Cause of Rising Health Care Costs
        Table 40–1. Causes of increasing health care costs.
      3. Cost Shifting
        Figure 40–3. Impact of cost shifting on business health care costs.
    B. Disability Management
        Figure 40–4. Increasing proportion of disability costs as percentage of total health care costs.
    C. Future Considerations
  II. Business Strategies in Health Care Management
    A. Restricting Benefits and Self-Insurance
    B. Cost Sharing
    C. Managing the Delivery of Health Care
      1. Utilization Review
      2. Managed Care
    D. Assessing Efforts at Cost Containment

Figure 40–5. Effectiveness of health programs in containing costs.
E. New Frontiers—Value Management
1. Prevention
2. Employee as Customer
3. Relationships with Suppliers
III. Opportunities for Occupational Physicians
Figure 40–6. Sectors of corporate physician's role.
Table 40–2. Three major role sectors for corporate medicine.
IV. Models of Physician Involvement in Health Care Management
A. Medical Liaison Model
1. Prevention and Health Promotion
2. Coordinating Chronic Disease
3. Convalescence
B. Medical Treatment Model
1. Personal Illness
2. Work-Related Conditions
C. Health Care Consultant Model
D. Health Management Leader
V. Summary
VI. References
VII. Appendix to Chapter 40: Getting Involved

KEY POINTS

- Business is concerned with costs of personal illness of employees and their dependents as well as the costs associated with work-related illness and injury.
- Most people with health insurance in the United States receive it through their employer. In 1990, 73% of all United States citizens with health insurance had coverage through their jobs. The majority of small employers provide health insurance.
- Employers have been actively trying to control health care costs by restricting benefits, sharing the cost with employees, and managing the delivery of health care.
- Utilization review (UR) allows payment only for services deemed necessary by the reviewer.
- Managed care programs began with health maintenance organizations (HMOs) paying premiums on a capitated, or per-person, basis. This model shifted the economic risk to the providers of care.
- Preferred provider organizations (PPOs) involve selected networks of doctors and hospitals that agree to accept discounts in prices and to cooperate with utilization review in exchange for an increased volume of patients.
- Contemporary programs to control health care costs include an increased focus on preventive interventions, involvement of the employee as a customer in the health care process, and working closely with suppliers to reduce variation in medical processes.
- Occupational physicians may be involved in management of health care costs by providing leadership in prevention of or convalescence from disease. In addition, the occupational physician has a role in referral of employees to the highest quality or most cost-effective community doctors.

QUESTIONS

*1. Which of the following statements regarding costs of health care in the United States is **false?***

A. The largest annual loss ever reported by a U.S. corporation was taken because of the estimated cost of health benefits.

B. A major component of the job descriptions of most occupational physicians employed by large corporations is control of total corporate expenditures for health care.
C. By 1991, health care costs in the United States totaled more than 14% of the gross national product (GNP).
D. Costs for personal illness of employees and dependents far outweigh the total costs associated with workers' compensation.
E. Health care management is evolving from an approach of pure cost containment to one of outcomes and quality measurement.

2. *Which of the following statements regarding financial incentives and health care costs is **false**?*

A. Under a fee-for-service insurance reimbursement arrangement, the physician bears no financial liability for ordering a medical test and the patient is insulated from its true cost.
B. When hospitals are paid on a cost-plus basis with the cost including capital expenditures, the financial incentive is in the direction of physical expansion and acquisition of new equipment.
C. Under fee-for-service reimbursement, physicians who perform more procedures are rewarded more than physicians who perform fewer procedures.
D. When physicians own ancillary medical service providers, such as clinical laboratories or radiology units, they may order more of those services than do physicians with no financial interest in the ancillary service.
E. The current interest in maximizing outpatient treatment is a direct result of high hospital occupancy rates.

3. *All of the following contribute to the current rise in health care costs incurred by companies **except**:*

A. cost shifting from the government to private employers.
B. technological developments in medical care.
C. capitated health care.
D. increasing costs of employee disabilities.
E. physician oversupply and specialization.

4. *Which of the following is **not** a strategy that businesses in the United States commonly use to control health care costs in their employees and dependents?*

A. Many businesses self-insure and, while doing so, they limit the maximum amount payable for certain high-cost illnesses, such as chronic psychiatric illnesses and infertility.
B. Many businesses have raised the deductibles and increased the percentage of medical treatment costs payable by the employee.
C. Some employers require the employee to obtain agreement on the part of the insurer that a hospital admission is necessary (preadmission certification).
D. Some employers have the insurer track inpatient services for appropriateness (concurrent review of inpatient services).
E. Many employers have discontinued insuring outpatient treatment on the grounds that it is associated with less quality assurance than is in-hospital treatment.

5. *Which of the following statements regarding employers' assessment of health care cost containment is true?*

A. Cost-containment efforts in the 1980s have exceeded expectations.

B. Increased cost sharing has helped reduce the rate of rise in health care costs.
C. Mandatory second opinions for elective surgery have reduced surgical procedures by over 40%.
D. Utilization review (UR) is typically regarded as helpful and as expediting needed patient care.
E. In the United States, rates of surgical treatment for common conditions, such as hysterectomies and coronary artery bypass grafts, are similar in big cities with tertiary care medical facilities, but vary widely in smaller cities and rural areas.

REFERENCES

Greenfield S, et al. Variations in resource utilization among medical specialties and systems of care: results from the Medical Outcomes Study. *J.A.M.A.* 267:1624, 1992.

Williams SJ, Torreas PR, eds. *Introduction to health services.* Albany, NY: Delmar, 1988.

The 1991 national executive poll on health care costs and benefits. *Business and Health* September 1991:62–68.

Section 4 Answers

CHAPTER 31 ANSWERS

1. The answer is D. (Reference: p. 447)

A 1991 Supreme Court decision (*International Union v. Johnson Controls,* 1991) does not allow employers to keep pregnant or fertile women from working in jobs that may injure a fetus and cause an adverse reproductive outcome. Rather, employees decide as individuals whether they will perform potentially hazardous jobs after receiving information on potential risks.

2. The answer is C. (Reference: p. 448)

Sexual differentiation begins about 7 weeks after conception and is completed by the fourth month in the male. FSH acts on the Sertoli cells in the testes to produce the release of a second hormone, LH, from the hypothalamic-pituitary axis. LH stimulates the testicular Leydig cells to produce testosterone. Although males and females have identical FSH and LH, it is the hormonal effects on six-specific target cells that produce sexual differentiation.

In adult men, the high rate of cell division during the 70 to 80 days of spermatogenesis makes this process susceptible to adverse influences. Spermatogonia undergo mitosis into spermatocytes; spermatids are produced by further cell division through meiosis and mature into the characteristic head and tail shape of sperm. Normal sperm production is about 20 to 350 million per day, with human ejaculate containing from 50 to 150 million per milliliter. Less than 20 million sperm per milliliter is considered to be clinical infertility (Radike, 1985). Fertility criteria have been defined as greater than 40% motile sperm, greater than 20 million sperm per milliliter of semen (normal sperm count is approximately 40–60 million/ml), and greater than 70% normal morphology (McLeod and Ving, 1979).

The entire complement of ova are present at birth, and their number gradually decreases with age. Only about 400 mature ova are released during ovulation in a lifetime.

3. The answer is D. (Reference: p. 449)

The potential interferences with the reproductive process are several. A healthy baby is the normal outcome if a healthy sperm fertilizes a healthy ovum that passes unimpeded through the fallopian tubes, implants in the uterus, develops normal organs, and grows to term. Interference with this basic process can occur with a change in libido or in the following steps, each an example of an interfering exposure:

1. The production of sperm.
2. The production of ova.
3. The fertilized ovum may not pass through the fallopian tube to the uterus.
4. The fertilized ovum may not implant in the uterus.
5. The embryo may be affected as its tissues differentiate or its organs develop.
6. The fetus may not grow normally, resulting in spontaneous abortions, stillbirths, or premature births.

4. The answer is A. (Reference: pp. 449, 450)

An agent or factor that causes physical birth defects or malformations in the developing embryo is termed a teratogen. The effects of a teratogen are dose related: A high dose is embryolethal, a moderate dose produces a defect, while a low dose may produce no effect. Teratogens are substances that produce birth defects or congenital malformations without producing toxicity in the mother. If a birth defect results from maternal toxicity, the defect may be caused by the toxic effects on the mother rather than a direct manifestation of the substance itself. The type of defect or malformation also depends on the day(s) during the period of organogenesis that exposure to the teratogen occurred.

General principles (American Medical Association Council on Scientific Affairs, 1985) of teratology are the following:

1. Susceptibility to teratogenesis depends on the genotype of the conceptus and the manner in which the genotype interacts with environmental factors.
2. Susceptibility to teratogenic agents varies with the developing stage of the fetus at the time of exposure.
3. Teratogenic agents act through specific mechanisms on developing cells and tissues, thus initiating abnormal embryogenesis.
4. The final manifestation of abnormal development is malformation, growth retardation, functional disorder, or death.
5. The access of adverse environmental influences to developing tissues depends on the nature of the influences (agents).
6. Manifestations of abnormal development increase from no effect to the totally lethal level as the dosage increases.

5. The answer is E. (Reference: Table 31–4)

6. The answer is E. (Reference: pp. 453, 457)

Items of importance to reproductive studies on test animals include:
1. Species. Studies on humans, nonhuman primates, and nonprimates may show marked variations in the rate of biotransformation. For example, the amount of phenylacetic acid excreted in the urine after conjugation to glutamine is almost 100% in humans, 30% to 90% in nonhuman primates, and none in nonprimates (O'Flaherty, 1985).
2. Dose-response. Measurable responses increase as the dosage frequency, duration, and intensity increase. Accurate dosage data are necessary to correlate dosage levels to the adverse outcome responses. For example, the concentration of a substance in parts per million (ppm) in a test animal's drinking water or feed may be known, but because the amount of water or feed the animal actually consumed may not be known, the total dose ingested is unknown. Higher doses in water or feed produce maternal toxicity and subsequent decreased maternal intake, which alters the dose delivered to the embryo or fetus. This altered dose cannot be accurately correlated to a response. A useful maximal dosage end point to determine whether the substance has an effect on the embryo or fetus is the dosage just below that which produces maternal toxicity.

Table 31–4. *Potentially confounding factors for a number of adverse reproductive effects*

Adverse reproductive effect	Potentially confounding factors
Impaired spermatogenesis	Surgical procedures such as vasectomy; diseases and illnesses such as varicocele, fever, mumps, and diabetes; certain therapeutic drugs
Reduced fertility	Contraceptive use
Spontaneous abortion	Maternal age, cigarette smoking, alcohol consumption, history of spontaneous abortions
Low birth weight	Race, cigarette smoking, parity, maternal nutrition
Birth defects: e.g., Down syndrome, neural tube defects	Maternal age, ethnic factors

Source: From Nisbet ICT, Karch NJ. *Chemical hazards to human reproduction.* Park Ridge, NJ: Noyes Data Corp., 1983, p. 44.

3. Route of administration. The skin or dermal exposure LD_{50} of many substances is about 10 times that for ingestion, and ingestion itself is about 10 times that for intravenous exposure. Occupational exposures occur frequently through the lung or inhalation route. Inhalation is a more efficient route of exposure than all others except intravenous.
4. Period of the reproductive process during which the animal is exposed to the substance. The first day of gestation may be referred to as day 0 or day 1, which introduces 1 day of error, a factor that becomes important during extrapolation of animal effects to humans. For example, a heart defect in animals is often assumed to produce a heart defect in humans when exposure occurs during the appropriate period of heart organogenesis.
5. Summary of effects. Adverse effects are generally described, along with a test of statistical significance. Often little consideration is given to biologic significance.

7. The answer is B. (Reference: p. 457)

Route of administration: see note in answer to question 6, above.

8. The answer is D. (Reference: p. 458, Table 31–6, Figure 31–2)

Some physicians respond to the woman who asks, "Will compound X hurt my baby?" by writing "No chemical use allowed" on a slip that is returned to the place of

Table 31–6. *Guidelines for continuation of various job tasks during pregnancy*

Job task	Week of gestation
Secretarial and light clerical	40
Professional and managerial	40
Sitting with light tasks	
Prolonged (more than 4 hours)	40
Intermittent	40
Standing	
Prolonged (more than 4 hours)	24
Intermittent	
More than 30 minutes per hour	32
Less than 30 minutes per hour	40
Stooping and bending below knee level	
Repetitive (more than 10 times per hour)	20
Intermittent	
2 to 20 times per hour	28
Less than 2 times per hour	40
Climbing	
Vertical ladders and poles	
Repetitive (4 or more times per 8-hour shift)	20
Intermittent (less than 4 times per 8-hour shift)	28
Stairs	
Repetitive (4 or more times per 8-hour shift)	28
Intermittent (less than 4 times per 8-hour shift)	40
Lifting	
Repetitive	
Less than 25 lb	40
25 to 50 lb	24
More than 50 lb	20
Intermittent	
Less than 25 lb	40
25 to 50 lb	40
More than 50 lb	30

Source: From American Medical Association Council on Scientific Affairs. Effect of pregnancy on work performance. *J.A.M.A.* 251:1995, 1984. Copyright 1984. American Medical Association.

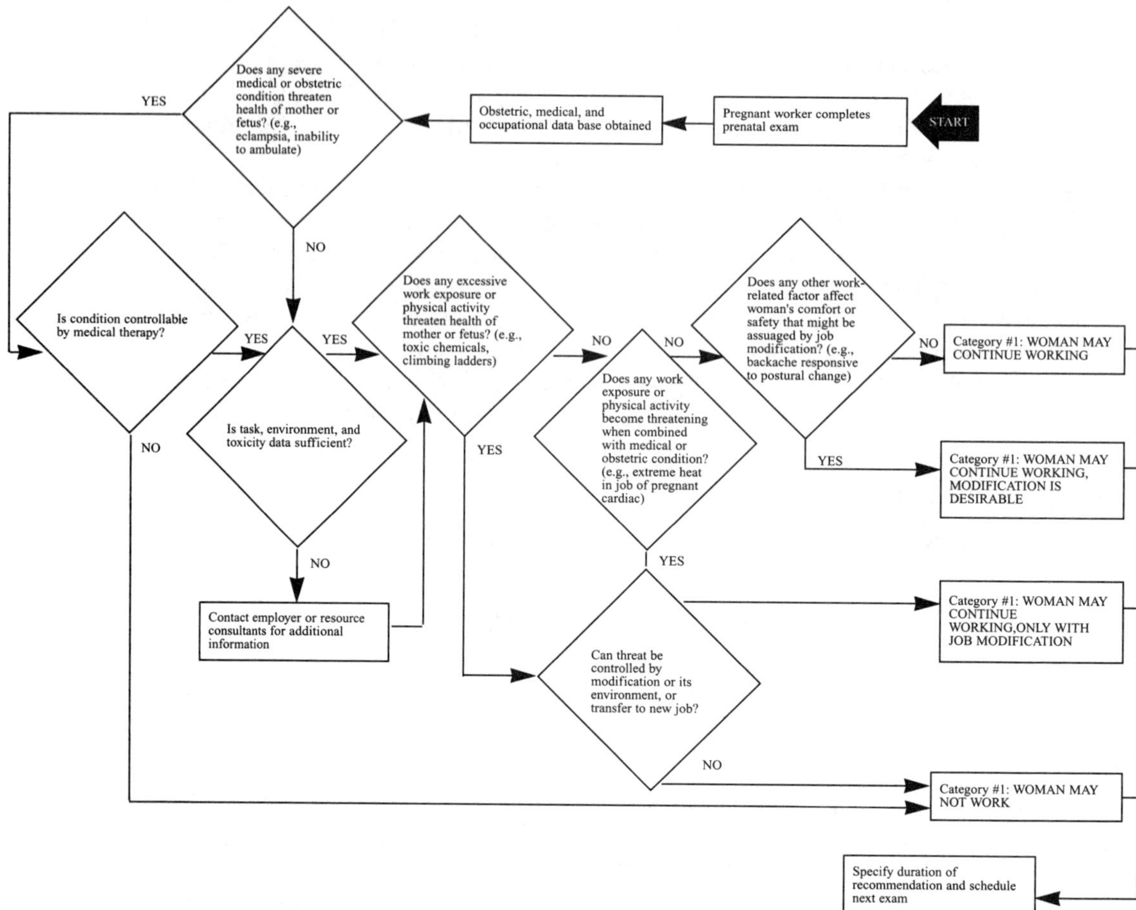

Figure 31–2. Algorithm for medical management of the pregnant worker. (From United States Department of Health and Human Services. Guidelines on Pregnancy and Work. NIOSH Publication no. 78-118, 1977, p. 14.)

employment. Unfortunately, this blanket response may needlessly heighten the patient's charged emotions and create volatile workplace situations and employee relations problems. This reflex-type response overlooks the myriad chemicals present in the home environment, in addition to neglecting a critical review of available information. Guidelines and methods for setting policy (Bond, 1986; Logan, 1986) and for determining if an individual may work in a job have been proposed (Fig. 31–2).

CHAPTER 32 ANSWERS

1. The answer is D. (Reference: p. 465)

Health promotion is now recognized as an important part of the practice of occupational health, as shown by the number of work sites with health promotion activities. This integration of activities is evidenced in the findings of the 1992 national survey, conducted by the United States Office of Disease Prevention and Health Promotion, documenting that 81% of work sites with 50 or more employees offer at least one health promotion activity, as compared to 65% of work sites in 1985. This growth since 1985, and the challenge for future growth of work-site health promotion, is certainly not born exclusively of established national goals. It is driven by the desire of employers to manage health care costs, impact absence, and contribute to the health and well-being of their human resources.

2. The answer is B. (Reference: p. 465)

Comprehensive programs give equal emphasis to establishing management support for health promotion activities, building a health-supporting work environment, fostering health activities as a viable business strategy, and helping employees identify health risks and behaviors in order to determine ways to change and improve.

3. The answer is B. (Reference: pp. 467–468)

At the outset of planning, a clear description of the expectations of the health promotion program is most essential.

Employee assessments, taking the form of surveys and focus groups, are a good place to begin. The goal is to understand the wants and needs of the population, as well as the ethnic, cultural, social, and organizational characteristics.

Management interviews gather another perspective, that of the leadership and supervision in the company. It is critical that the needs of the business are understood and that the issues of managers are taken into consideration.

Health care cost data, illness/injury absence data, and demographic data should be used to determine the prominent disease categories that are driving costs, and for which groups of employees.

Finally, data from health risk appraisals (HRA) can be used to develop and aggregate a view of population, information that is essential to program planning.

4. The answer is C. (Reference: p. 468)

Some of the more popular programs offered in the business setting: smoking cessation, exercise/aerobics, nutrition/cholesterol/weight management, blood pressure control, stress management, employee assistance programs, and preventive examinations.

5. The answer is B. (Reference: p. 473)

The evaluation component should be developed at the beginning of the program when considering the interests of all stakeholders. Determinations about data points and intervals are elements of the evaluation component. Without an evaluation design, the effects of a health promotion program will not be systematically measured, and the ability to justify continuing a program may be lost.

CHAPTER 33 ANSWERS

1. The answer is B. (Reference: p. 480)

The occupational history is the clinical tool used to elicit and organize information about the workplace for any thorough diagnostic evaluation.

A basic occupational history includes the following:

1. Description of current and recent work, including longest held job and years worked in each position.
2. Report of any exposure to chemicals, dusts, or fumes, including type, intensity, and duration; and information from manufacturers, employers, and Material Safety Data Sheets (MSDS).
3. Relationship of symptoms to periods away from work (e.g., weekends, holidays, vacations, or other absence) and to changes in work schedule.
4. Description of any change in work activities, production quotas, work processes, or other work routine preceding or coinciding with the development of symptoms.
5. Occurrence of similar symptoms or illness in co-workers.
6. The patient's opinion regarding the relationship of illness to work and reasons supporting the opinion.
7. History of use of substances in avocational activities and their relationship to symptoms or illness.
8. Contact with workplace of work-site visit.

2. The answer is D. (Reference: p. 483)

The occupational history should be taken in sufficient detail to identify the type, intensity, and duration of exposure to materials. If specific exposure information is not known, description of work activities and processes may be an adequate substitute.

3. The answer is E. (Reference: p. 483)

Manufacturers of substances may be able to provide information on chemical formulations and toxicity.

A number of texts on industrial processes are useful for understanding work activities, potential for exposures, and chemical or physical agents that should be considered as potential causes of disease.

Review of MSDS can yield clues for further investigation.

A number of government agencies provide information on commercial substances and their effect on health. For example, the National Institute for Occupational Safety and Health (NIOSH) has regional offices that can provide current information.

The Index Medicus and National Library of Medicine computerized literature searches (e.g., MEDLINE, TOXLINE) are becoming routine tools in this stage of the information-gathering process.

4. The answer is A. (Reference: p. 482)

Case reports of clusters of tumors of unusual type or at unusual anatomic sites have led to identification of occupational carcinogens. In addition to peculiar cancers, clusters of people with unusual symptoms, such as difficulty in urinating among foam workers exposed to a newly introduced catalyst, dimethylaminopropionitrile (Kreiss et al., 1980), and clusters of people with unusual illness (e.g., aspermia in workers exposed to the nematocide dibromochloropropane (Whorton et al., 1977)) in groups sharing work experiences have led to case reports of new relationships between exposure and disease.

5. The answer is B. (Reference: pp. 486, 487)

Case reports in occupational medicine that contribute most to new and useful knowledge will usually be one of the following:

the unique case
a new association of an illness with exposure to a material or other stressor
an unexpected course of an illness
a case that clarifies pathophysiology

CHAPTER 34 ANSWERS

1. The answer is E. (Reference: p. 491)

The mission, goals, and objectives of the occupational health program (OHP) should be congruent with and support the mission, goals, and objectives of the organization.

In the face of increasing medical care costs and significant questions about the value received for these massive outlays, occupational physicians are becoming more involved in benefits redesign and medical management.

Adverse health effects from the workplace should be prevented by medical surveillance and control of hazardous exposures.

2. The answer is E. (Reference: p. 492)

Employers are prohibited from asking a variety of medical questions that are not directly related to the functional requirements of the job.

3. The answer is A. (Reference: pp. 493, 494)

One example of clinical surveillance is early detection of CTDs, also known as repetitive strain injuries, which are typically preceded by symptoms of muscle or tendon overuse that may progress to permanent injury. The majority of cases filed under workers' compensation as carpal tunnel syndrome and other CTDs are precursor inflammation and pain syndromes, rather than disorders that meet the diagnostic criteria for carpal tunnel syndrome or other such disorders. Alert practitioners in regular contact with workers in repetitive motion jobs can screen for the discomfort that precedes disabling tendonitis, rotator cuff syndrome, and other CTDs, and recommend job redesign or other preventive interventions.

4. The answer is D. (Reference: p. 494)

A key duty of the occupational health professional is to monitor health-related data on members of the work force exposed to chemical, radiation, and other physical hazards and to compare the values for exposed and unexposed groups periodically. If an increased prevalence of abnormal laboratory values or symptoms is detected in an exposed group, the exposure should be quantified and controlled through engineering measures, administrative efforts (i.e., rotating employees), or personal protective equipment, in that order. The economic value of this type of service depends on the cost of the disease avoided, which can be computed for a population of workers if the probability of illness is known for various levels of exposure.

5. The answer is D. (Reference: p. 495)

Immunization is an example of primary prevention resulting from a surveillance program. Workers in health care facilities, prisons, and waste disposal and sanitation are at high risk of hepatitis, influenza, and other blood-, body fluid–, or aerosol-borne diseases. The economic benefit of immunization of workers in these critical community services against influenza (Recommendations of the Immunization Practice Advisory Committee, 1985) and hepatitis B (Recommendations for Protection against Viral Hepatitis, 1985) has been demonstrated. Health care workers should also be primarily immunized against hepatitis B.

6. The answer is C. (Reference: p. 497)

EAPs provide savings by early intervention in mental health problems, which can prevent hospitalization and long-term illness. Nonproductive conflicts between employees and supervisors can be resolved early, as can performance problems due to stress or substance abuse (Bureau of National Affairs, 1986). It should be noted that performance problems not related to an illness or injury are the province of the supervisor and not occupational health professionals, who should be careful to separate the two issues.

CHAPTER 35 ANSWERS

1. The answer is C. (Reference: p. 510)

In a separate report, the IOM recommended that all primary care physicians be able to identify possible occupationally or environmentally induced conditions and make appropriate referrals for follow-up (Institute of Medicine, 1988). The fund of knowledge required to meet such a standard of care included familiarity with principles of preventive medicine as well as occupational and environmental medicine, clinical skills in occupational history taking, a basic knowledge of common occupational and environmental diseases, and an understanding of the United States regulatory system and workers' compensation system.

2. The answer is B. (Reference: p. 510)

Recognizing this changing practice climate, the ACGME now requires some element of occupational medicine training in accredited family medicine training programs (AMA, 1992). Other boards and specialty areas such as internal medicine are likely to follow. National initiatives such as the Academic Award in Occupational/Environmental Medicine by the National Institute of Environmental Health Sciences (NIEHS) are aimed at developing occupational and environmental medicine faculty and curricula for medical schools to expose students to the field at an early stage in their medical education.

3. The answer is E. (Reference: p. 511)

The most fundamental distinction is that occupational and environmental medicine is a specialty that focuses on the prevention of illness and injury at work.

To competently deliver occupational medical services, one must be more than just a good clinician. In most private practices, the clinician waits for the patient to come to the clinic with certain symptoms, makes a diagnosis, and prescribes a course of treatment. The occupational medicine physician deals primarily with a healthy work force, and often focuses on medical surveillance of workers to identify potentially hazardous exposures at a stage when disease can be prevented.

4. The answer is A. (Reference: p. 511)

Funding for occupational medicine residency training, although derived from a variety of sources, faces serious shortages if training centers are to fill the recognized void of specialists. NIOSH provides some degree of funding to most training programs through the ERCs and program training grants. However, such grants generally cover only a portion of training costs. Residency programs also rely on scholarships, corporate grants, income from consultative and clinical services, and a variety of innovative funding mechanisms. A significant source of scholarship support is the Occupational Physician's Scholarship Fund established with corporate support by the ACOEM.

5. The answer is C. (Reference: p. 512)

In 1992, 37 residency training programs in occupational medicine were accredited by the ACGME in the United States, an increase from 25 in 1986 (AMA, 1992). Occupational medicine residencies vary widely in size (ranging from 1 to over 10 residents). Nationwide, approximately 75 to 100 physicians graduate each year. The academic and clinical focus varies from program to program, but all provide trainees with the fundamental academic and practical knowledge to practice occupational medicine in a variety of settings.

6. The answer is D. (Reference: p. 513)

The ACOEM sponsors seminars and courses related to the specialty. In addition to postgraduate seminars and courses offered at the national meetings in the spring and fall of each year, the college periodically sponsors 1- or 2-day courses of particular interest to practitioners. Recent examples include medical review officer (MRO) courses and seminars on the Americans with Disabilities Act (ADA). The ACOEM also offers the basic curriculum, a structured series of three 2-day segments designed to provide the nonoccupational medicine specialist with useful information and an introduction to occupational and environmental medicine.

CHAPTER 36 ANSWERS

1. The answer is D. (Reference: p. 518)

There are two basic uses of computers in occupational medical practice. The first is office automation involving the use of software programs for word processing, spreadsheet, project planning, graphics, client contact, communication, personal assistance, computer utilities and similar functions.

Occupational medical applications are the second use, with a growing number of database management systems being tailored to the occupational health user. Some are focused on a single purpose (e.g., generating random numbers for drug testing or preparing the Occupational Safety and Health Administration [OSHA] report of first injury). Others handle multiple purposes and are usually described as an occupational health information system (OHIS).

2. The answer is C. (Reference: p. 519)

Computers are quickly becoming essential management tools with valued applications in all aspects of OM. The use of a successful OHIS can significantly improve an organization's ability to achieve its goals through (1) improved efficiency and productivity, (2) enhanced quality and decision making, (3) regulatory compliance and litigation assistance, and (4) the ability to inexpensively create additional supplemental and new services.

3. The answer is E. (Reference: p. 524)

One of the most important components of an OHIS system—indeed, perhaps the most important component—is support of the office staff in the pursuit of everyday tasks. Document preparation (word processing), spreadsheets, contact and time managers, project time lines, and electronic mail are all important parts of general office automation support. Without integration of these functions, the OHIS may not be used. Most users already have these support programs on their desktop computers, and they do not want to (1) learn new systems, (2) have two computers on their desk, or (3) leave their desk in order to do their job.

4. The answer is D. (Reference: p. 525)

Separate medical records are often kept by EAP counselors. Automated EAP systems or EAP components of an OHIS with restricted access allow generation of activity reports, tracking and follow-up of individuals, and group reporting for evaluation purposes.

CHAPTER 37 ANSWERS

1. The answer is B. (Reference: p. 538)

At virtually any manufacturing facility employing ten workers or more, some fundamental training requirements are mandatory. These requirements range from fire protection to respirator use, hearing, process safety management, and medical services, as well as related duties for contractors, the mechanical integrity of equipment, and appropriate prevention signs and tags.

2. The answer is E. (Reference: p. 539)

Employers are held accountable by OSHA to ensure that people who need to wear respirators in the course of their work are medically certified. Although OSHA has considered implementing a standard on the use of personal protective equipment, there are presently no universal medical criteria to which the physician decision-making process must adhere. It is up to the judgment of the examining physician as to whether a person can be medically cleared for respirator use.

3. The answer is E. (Reference: p. 539)

The employer shall institute a training program for all employees who are exposed to noise at or above an 8-hour TWA of 85 dB, and shall ensure employee participation in such a program. The training program shall be repeated yearly for each employee included in the hearing conservation program. The training program should inform the employee about (1) the effects of noise on hearing; (2) the purpose of hearing protectors, as well as the advantages, disadvantages, and attenuation of various types and instructions on selection, fitting, use, and care; and (3) the purpose of audiometric testing and an explanation of the test procedure.

4. The answer is C. (Reference: p. 540)

The employer shall ensure the ready availability of medical personnel for advise and consultation on matters of plant health.

In the absence of an infirmary, clinic, or hospital in close proximity to the workplace, a person or persons shall be adequately trained to render first aid. First-aid supplies approved by the consulting physician shall be readily available. Where the eyes or body of any person may be exposed to injurious corrosive materials, suitable facilities for quick drenching or flushing of the eyes and body shall be provided within the work area for immediate emergency use.

5. The answer is D. (Reference: p. 541)

In November 1983, OSHA promulgated the Hazard Communication Standard, a regulation covering a broad range of chemical hazards. This standard contains specific provisions regarding the evaluation of health hazards, labeling of containers, use of chemical information sheets (MSDSs), and training of employees. Also known as HazCom, the standard originally applied only to chemical manufacturers, importers, and distributors, but was later expanded to cover many additional employers. Presently, all companies and employers that handle any hazardous substance in any form are required to comply with the standard (O'Neill et al., 1988).

6. The answer is C. (Reference: p. 541)

Material Safety Data Sheets are a foundation of a successful safety and health program. They provide information that can be used during employee training and chemical exposure emergencies; they also give vital information to medical professionals caring for the affected employee. They inform employees of the health hazards of chemicals with which they are working and let them know what situations can produce explosion and decomposition hazards. Their purpose is to communicate critical facts about working safely with the material (Garbo et al., 1988).

7. The answer is B. (Reference: p. 542, Table 37–1)

OSHA published the final rule of its laboratory standard, Occupational Exposures to Hazardous Chemicals in Laboratories, in the January 31, 1990, Federal Register (29 CFR 1919.1450).

The standard applies to all laboratories that use hazardous chemicals in accordance with the definition, chemical for which there is statistical significant evidence based on at least one study conducted in accordance with established scientific principles that acute or chronic health effects may occur in exposed employees (Kilby, 1990). This would include chemicals that are carcinogens, toxic or highly toxic agents, reproductive toxins, irritants, corrosives, sensitizers, hepatotoxins, nephrotoxins, neurotoxins, agents that affect the hematopoietic system, and agents that damage the lungs, skin, eyes, or mucous membranes. This is further detailed in the Hazard Communication Standard, and outlined in Table 37–1.

Table 37–1. *Toxins and their effects*

Toxin category	Definition	Signs/symptoms	Chemicals
Hepatoxin	Chemical that produces liver damage	Jaundice; liver enlargement	Carbon tetrachloride; nitrosamines
Nephrotoxin	Chemical that produces kidney damage	Edema; proteinuria	Halogenated hydrocarbons; uranium
Neurotoxin	Chemical that produces its primary toxic effects on the nervous system	Narcosis; behavioral changes; decreases in motor function	Mercury; carbon disulfide
Agents that act on the blood or hematopoietic system	Chemicals that decrease hemoglobin function; deprive the body tissue of oxygen	Cyanosis; loss of consciousness	Carbon monoxide; cyanide
Agents that damage the lung	Chemicals that irritate or damage the pulmonary tissue	Cough; tightness in chest; shortness of breath	Silica; asbestos
Reproductive toxin	Chemical that affects the reproductive capabilities, including chromosomal damage (mutations) and effects on the fetus (teratogenesis)	Birth defects; sterility	Lead; dibromodichloropropane (DBCP)
Cutaneous hazard	Chemical that affects the dermal layer of the body	Defatting of the skin; rashes; irritation	Ketones; chlorinated compounds
Eye hazard	Chemical that affects the eye or visual capacity	Conjunctivitis; corneal damage	Organic solvents; acids

CHAPTER 38 ANSWERS

1. The answer is E. (Reference: p. 549)

The occupational medicine physician can best serve employees internationally by providing appropriate protocols for common medical problems, baseline medical examinations, and country protocols for diseases that local physicians will treat. Working with the human resources department in developing guidelines for employee selection is another useful contribution that an occupational physician can make.

2. The answer is D. (Reference: pp. 550, 553)

Kits are most effective if they are specific for the person's needs. A small amount of certain medications may be included in the medical kit for conditions that do not necessitate long-term treatment. Travelers should carry a letter signed by a physician on letterhead or prescription pad indicating the need for the medications and medical equipment contained in the medical kit. These papers should be kept with the medical kit. ("This patient has been required to carry the following medication for medical reasons.") This measure will prevent the person from embarrassing and potentially long-term delays at international borders by curious customs agents. If routine medication is used, it is wise to state the patient's major health-related problems and the medication dosage on a prescription pad.

3. The answer is B. (Reference: p. 555)

For the traveler to the world's capitals, bottled water is usually available. You will rarely see local Parisians or Dubliners drinking tap water. Although usually safe, faulty medieval water pipes in certain sections of otherwise highly advanced cities allow for contamination. Travelers should be reminded to remove the plastic seal on any bottle sold as purified water. Carbonated water gives yet one more guarantee that the bottled water has not been tampered with. Heating water to 62°C for 10 minutes is sufficient to eliminate all strains of bacteria. Adding iodine or chlorine and allowing the water to sit for 30 minutes will disinfect the filtered water. Sediments should be filtered before adding the iodine or chlorine to ensure complete killing of the bacteria, parasites, worm larvae, and particularly viruses.

4. The answer is D. (Reference: p. 556)

There are several ways of managing jet lag. For the fastidious person who has time to plan meals 3 days before travel, a diet that alternates a feast and fast of high carbohydrates and high proteins is available. Unfortunately, most travelers cannot adhere to this diet in a way that makes it effective. On a dietary basis, however, one may modify, to some extent, the symptoms of jet lag by eating a high-carbohydrate dinner the night before travel and, on the trip, eating salads, fruit plates, and other light dishes. Similarly, the employee should drink plenty of fluids before and during the air travel to reduce both jet lag and air travel fatigue. Alcohol before or during the trip should be avoided because it increases the effects of jet lag and suppresses the rapid eye movement (REM) phase of sleep, the most critical component of the sleep cycle.

5. The answer is D. (Reference: p. 557)

For the traveler who has had contact with locals in a factory, health care facility, or private home, or had questionable dietary intake, and for those who may have reduced resistance to disease, routine screening is often recommended. Ancillary testing may vary from a complete blood count (CBC), erythrocyte sedimentation rate (ESR), and chemistry panel to urinalysis, tuberculin skin test, and stool for ova, parasites, and the culture. These tests should be modified based on the countries visited and the person's symptoms. Serologic screening for hepatitis, schistosomiasis, filariasis, or dengue fever may be indicated (Gustatsson, 1987; Warren, 1985). Certain tropically acquired diseases may remain latent for extended periods of time.

6. The answer is E. (Reference: pp. 557, 558)

If the traveler is vigilant and meticulous in eating and drinking, as the CDC suggests, prophylactic antibiotics are not necessary. For the short-term visit to certain countries, such as North Americans traveling to Mexico, prophylactic antibiotics may be appropriate (i.e., doxycycline, 100 mg/day, or trimethoprim/sulfamethoxazole, 1 tablet/day) (Steffan et al., 1988). Prophylaxis and/or treatment of simple traveler's diarrhea can be achieved with bismuth-salicylate (Pepto-Bismol), 2 tablets q.i.d.. This treatment and prophylaxis is usually effective.

7. The answer is D. (Reference: p. 558)

AIDS has spread rapidly in Asia, West and East Africa, Latin America, and parts of Europe within the heterosexual population. Since sexual contact is the major route of HIV infection in the traveler, people should be advised about safe sex practices, especially with persons in whom the HIV infection status is unknown.

CHAPTER 39 ANSWERS

1. The answer is D. (Reference: p. 564)

Workers' compensation management has become more visible in recent years because of an increase in the number of lost workdays per 100 employees and a rapid increase in the cost of both wage replacement and medical treatment. Wage replacement costs are increasing at almost twice the rate of the general wage index, and medical care costs are rising two to three times faster than the medical consumer price index. Effective management of workers' compensation provides a challenge to the administrative and clinical skills of the occupational physician. The effort, however, can benefit both the injured worker with more effective medical care and the employer by increasing availability for work and decreasing unnecessary costs.

2. The answer is D. (Reference: p. 565)

Another ANSI coding scheme classifies injuries by the part of the body that was injured. Back injuries, which are debatably injuries in the sense that there is infrequently a discrete acute event involved, and which may be due to nonwork events or cumulative trauma, have been the largest category of body parts injured for several years, accounting for 22% of cases and 31% of compensation costs.

3. The answer is B. (Reference: p. 564)

The top five occupational causes of deaths are motor vehicle accidents (35.5%), falls (12.7%), electric current accidents (3.6%), burns (3.5%), and noningestive poisoning (3.5%).

4. The answer is E. (Reference: p. 568)

All industrial and most service employment is covered by workers' compensation statutes; however, farm labor, domestic service and casual employees are usually exempted from the laws.

The federal Social Security Disability Program pays benefits to disabled workers under the age of 65 when disability is expected to last 12 months or longer or results in death. Benefits are financed by the federal Social Security Tax.

There is considerable dispute about the adequacy of workers' compensation coverage. In 1972, the National Commission on State Workers' Compensation Laws recommended 84 revisions in state systems to improve compensation, make the state laws more consistent, and remove certain inequities. However, most states have not completed these recommendations, 19 of which were considered essential.

5. The answer is C. (Reference: pp. 569, 570)

The National Council on Compensation Insurance (National Council on Compensation Insurance, 1992) estimated that $60 billion was paid out in 1991 for wage replacement, administrative and legal costs, and medical costs.

The average medical cost per case for workers' compensation payments now exceeds $6,000.

It is widely believed that there is extensive cost shifting from Medicare, Medicaid, and other government programs, as well as from private insurance, because cost-containment programs have succeeded in those areas but have not been widely used in workers' compensation.

There is also a belief that all medical bills must be paid, although, in fact, few statutes or regulations make that statement. The correct statement is that medically necessary care must be reimbursed.

6. The answer is C. (Reference: p. 570)

Benefits are provided for wage replacement, medical and legal expenses, and permanent impairment. Lump-sum compensation is paid for certain scheduled physical damage or loss of function such as the loss of a body part, whereas medical and wage replacement payments are made whenever there is a wage loss related to work.

When there is lost time, income replacement payments are made on a weekly basis according to a formula expressed as a percentage of wages. Most states have maximum and minimum limits; some states limit the total number of weeks payable.

7. The answer is E. (Reference: p. 572)

With reductions in group health benefits, there has been a tendency to ascribe injuries to the work site, since workers' compensation will pay 100% of the medical bills and provide wage replacement. As group health benefits continue to be reduced or are eliminated by smaller employers, this incentive to use the workers' compensation system is expected to increase.

8. The answer is C. (Reference: p. 573)

There is a clear need for proactive medical management of workers' compensation cases because of the wide variations in the quality and quantity of medical care, and the absence of medical expertise under the present property and casualty insurance framework. The need for standards and criteria is made more urgent by the fact that many of the current major categories of occupational illness or injury are nonspecific subjective complaints, such as back and wrist pain, that can only be effectively managed with carefully constructed criteria and constant reference to physical signs.

For example, it has been demonstrated repeatedly that the average recovery time for uncomplicated low back pain is 2 days of bed rest and 8 days of partial disability before complete return to function (Deyo et al., 1986). However, comparison of a survey by the American College of Occupational and Environmental Medicine (unpublished data now used by Beech Street, Inc.) and several other consensus panels (Doyle et al., 1990; Harris et al., 1989; Reed, 1990) revealed that while the average length of time absent from work for both back pain and wrist pain is in the range of 4 to 15 weeks, the expert consensus was 1 to 3 weeks.

CHAPTER 40 ANSWERS

1. The answer is B. (Reference: p. 581)

Although there has been limited involvement with disability costs associated with work-related conditions, occupational doctors have had only a very minor role in the much greater cost problem associated with personal illness. This seems to be the result of a mutual reluctance, with occupational medicine largely perceiving health cost issues as outside its traditional scope of work-site health and safety, and business viewing physicians as having a trained incapacity to manage financial issues.

2. The answer is E. (Reference: p. 583)

The hospital industry for years has had an occupancy rate of approximately 70%, which has led to incentives both to have the empty beds filled and to raise prices to compensate for the unused equipment. Physician supply grew 40% between 1970 and 1987 (Harris JS, presented at ACOEM annual meeting, 1991), largely as a result of a taskforce report that had predicted a physician shortage. However, the predicted shortage was for primary care physicians in rural areas, and the new doctors largely became specialists in large metropolitan areas. Studies have clearly shown that health care costs increase directly with both oversupply and specialization (Greenfield et al., 1992).

3. The answer is C. (Reference: pp. 583, 584)

The paradoxical relationship between supply and demand in the health system, known as Roemer's law, is an important contributor to rising health care costs. It is characterized by a situation in which supply creates demand, the reverse of classic economic market theory.

In the health care system, this is due to many factors: an infinite desire for health, a highly technical field that makes it difficult for an individual to act as an informed consumer, and the aforementioned financing system, which disconnects the buyer from the payment (Williams and Torreas, 1988).

A further factor in the rise of health costs has been the astounding growth in high-technology medical procedures.

In addition to the factors listed in Table 40–1, business has faced the unique problem of cost shifting. As government increasingly controlled its health expenditures by statute (e.g., Medicare price freezes and hospital prospective payment), the providers of care shifted the burden of payment to the private employers.

4. The answer is E. (Reference: pp. 586, 587)

The most popular forms of utilization review are preadmission certification and concurrent review of inpatient services. Both of these types of review seek to limit hospital days, as care delivered in this setting is the most expensive.

However, by the late 1970s it was evident that inpatient care was much more expensive than outpatient care, and that more procedures could safely be done in the outpatient setting, with considerable savings for the payer.

5. The answer is B. (Reference: p. 588)

Employers view increased cost sharing with employees as a successful intervention. In a 1990 poll, close to 50% of employers viewed this as an effective way to control health care costs (the 1991 national executive poll on health care costs and benefits, 1991).

Section 5

41

The Environment and Health

OBJECTIVES

- List causes of global warming
- Explain long-term effects anticipated as a result of ozone depletion
- Discuss causes and effects of acid rain

OUTLINE

I. Dimensions of the problem
   A. Atmospheric Changes
      1. Climate Change and the Greenhouse Effect
      2. Ozone Depletion and Ultraviolet Irradiation
      3. Acid Precipitation
      4. Population
   B. Sustainable Development
II. Implications for Physicians
III. References

KEY POINTS

- The degradation of the environment has become a major global problem, outstripping its local public health dimensions and becoming a serious threat. The implications of environmental trends for weather, human habitation, and food supply suggest serious trouble in years to come.
- The greenhouse effect contributes to stability of the world's temperature by allowing infrared radiation to reach the Earth's surface and by preventing the escape of radiant heat into space; this dual action maintains the biosphere within a temperature range conducive to life. As a result of industrial development, an increasing concentration of certain atmospheric gases are trapping too much infrared radiation, causing an increase in global temperature.
- The net effect of global warming may include more extremes of temperature with increased numbers of very hot days and a longer duration of heat waves. Ocean cur-

rents may be disrupted and anomalous flows of air could develop. This may increase the frequency and severity of violent weather disturbances such as hurricanes, tornadoes, typhoons, floods, and blizzards. The combination of these events could lead to food shortages because of the adverse effects of such weather on agriculture.

- Stratospheric depletion of ozone may increase exposure to ultraviolet (UV) radiation, which at the surface of the earth is most likely to result in damage to the skin, eyes, and possibly the immune system.
- Commercial sunscreens may be effective against UV-induced sunburn if they have a high enough sun protection factor for the exposure period, but their effectiveness against UV-induced cancer is unproven.
- Increased production and airborne transport of acidifying emissions from industrial sources, principally sulfates and nitrates, has caused increased acidity of soil and water. Acid precipitation is most detrimental to delicate aquatic ecosystems, marine biota, and some species of plants and trees.
- The world population is increasing at a rate that has outstripped our capacity to provide for them from the renewable resources of the planet.
- Sustainable development involves the establishment of an economic structure that ideally consumes only as much as the natural environment produces and emits only as much as the natural environment can absorb. This goal is accomplished by reducing consumption and the scale of economic development as well as by recycling materials.

QUESTIONS

1. What climatic change is most likely to be observed if current views of global warming are correct?

A. Paradoxical cooling because of cloud cover
B. Gradual prolonged successive summer heat waves
C. Imperceptible variations from existing weather conditions
D. Exaggerated extremes in temperature and chaotic local weather conditions
E. Uniform, drastic increases in temperature

2. The most likely health outcome from chlorofluorocarbon use and ozone depletion is

A. acute CFC toxicity.
B. increased frequency of opportunistic infections.
C. increased incidence of all cancers.
D. increased incidence of skin cancers.
E. reduction of ozone-associated respiratory irritation.

*3. Which of the following is **least** likely to affect human health via ecological change?*

A. Population growth
B. Sophisticated tertiary medical care
C. Technological change
D. Trade and importation of goods
E. Value systems in culture and religion

4. Which world region is at greatest human health risk as a result of multiple environmental changes?

A. Arctic and antarctic regions
B. Eastern hemisphere

C. Temperate regions
D. Tropical regions
E. Western hemisphere

5. Sustainable development involves

A. economic changes that reduce consumption.
B. economic changes that constantly replace in excess resources over use.
C. balancing consumption and production.
D. giving over production to community control.
E. linkage of production and corporate policy.

REFERENCES

Charman WN. Ocular hazards arising from depletion of the natural atmospheric ozone layer: a review. *Ophthalmic Physiol. Opt.* 10:333, 1990.

The environment and population growth: decade for action. Pop. Rep. (Population Information Program, The Johns Hopkins University) Special Issue, Series M (20), May 1992.

Henriksen T, et al. Ultraviolet radiation and skin cancer. Effect of an ozone layer depletion. *Photochem. Photobiol.* 51:578, 1990.

Kripke ML. Photoimmunology. *Photochem. Photobiol.* 52:919, 1990.

Longstreth J. Cutaneous malignant melanoma and ultraviolet radiation: a review. *Cancer Metastasis Rev.* 7:321, 1988.

Morison WL. Effects of ultraviolet radiation on the immune system in humans. *Photochem. Photobiol.* 50:515, 1989.

Olson CM. Increased outdoor recreation, diminished ozone layer pose ultraviolet radiation threat to eye. *J.A.M.A.* 261:1102, 1989.

Van Juijk FJGM. Effects of ultraviolet light on the eye: Role of protective glasses. *Environ. Health Perspect.* 96:177, 1991.

Vitasa BC, et al. Association of nonmelanoma skin cancer and actinic keratosis with cumulative solar ultraviolet exposure in Maryland watermen. *Cancer* 65:2881, 1990.

42

Environmental Medicine: The Regulatory Issues

OBJECTIVES

- List and explain the major environmental regulatory acts and agencies of the federal government
- Discuss the relationship between environmental regulation and the practice of environmental medicine

OUTLINE

KEY POINTS

- Environmental protection policies and laws create an expansive set of regulations to control pollution. Many of these regulations are oriented to minimize exposure by controlling emissions of categories of pollutants according to medium of exposure.
- Environmental regulations mirror public concern and its reflection of actual risk. As a result, regulations in the United States and other countries have been driven by a series of environmental issues, many of which arose from catastrophic situations.
- The Environmental Protection Agency (EPA) was established in 1970, and unified federal regulation of the environment. The EPA's charter included all media (air, water, and solid and hazardous waste).
- In 1970, the National Environmental Policy Act (NEPA) was established to promote concern for the environment by all federal agencies, and the Council of Environmental Quality (CEQ) was instituted.
- Other regulations that were passed included the Clean Air Act (CAA) and the Federal Water Pollution Control Act or Clean Water Act (CWA).
- In 1976, the Toxic Substances Control Act (TSCA) was passed in response to growing public concerns about the hazards of certain chemicals such as polychlorinated biphenyls (PCBs) and insecticides. In the same year, the Resource Conservation and Recovery Act (RCRA) was passed to regulate the disposal of solid and liquid hazardous waste.
- In 1980, the Comprehensive Environmental Response, Compensation, and Liability Act (CERCLA) was passed. This regulation addresses existing hazardous waste sites in the United States. It created the Superfund to address issues of adverse health effects from hazardous waste sites.
- The potential interfaces between environmental medicine and these regulations include (1) recognition of the database for correlating exposure to disease, (2) reporting requirements generated by environmental exposures, (3) knowledge of the regulatory system for environmental pollution, and (4) intervention strategies in environmentally induced disease or risk of disease.
- RCRA addresses the management of solid and liquid hazardous waste and is designed to minimize such waste by regulation of its transportation, storage, treatment, and disposal. It also addresses underground storage tanks by establishing design, monitoring, reporting, and removal requirements.
- CERCLA (Superfund) is designed to cover past hazardous waste activities, but also has reporting requirements for spills or other releases.
- In 1986, an amendment of the Superfund created the Emergency Planning and Community Right to Know Act (EPCRA). It is designed to make emergency planning entities aware of the presence of potentially hazardous substances through reporting requirements to state and local authorities.
- TSCA addresses the need to fully evaluate the potential toxicity and environmental impact of existing and new chemicals. A manufacturer (or importer) must notify the Office of Toxic Substances 90 days before producing or importing a new chemical substance. Such notification may prompt the need for additional testing. For existing chemicals, the act requires reporting of any significant adverse effects from animal or human studies or clinical cases that are not already known or reported.

QUESTIONS

1. Environmental regulations are

A. all federally mandated.
B. designed to prevent human disease.
C. designed to protect animals and plants.

D. only based in civil law.
E. pollutant specific.

2. *The review of testing of new commercial chemicals for potential toxicity primarily comes under the jurisdiction of the*

A. Department of Agriculture.
B. EPA.
C. NIEHS.
D. NIOSH.
E. OSHA.

3. *Environmental legislation frequently follows major catastrophic events. Community Right to Know legislation came in the aftermath of:*

A. Bhopal.
B. Love Canal.
C. Telluride.
D. Three Mile Island.
E. *Valdez* oil spill.

4. *Public access to air pollution information data is primarily mandated by the*

A. Comprehensive Environmental Response, Compensation and Liability Act (CERCLA).
B. Clean Air Act.
C. Emergency Planning and Community Right to Know Act (EPCRA).
D. Resource Conservation and Recovery Act (RCRA).
E. Toxic Substance Control Act (TSCA).

5. *Which of the following is **not** regulated by the Clean Water Act?*

A. Discharge permit programs
B. Grants for treatment facilities
C. Minimal effluent guidelines
D. Storage tank holdings
E. Storm water runoff

REFERENCES

Anderson FR, Mandelker DR. *Environmental protection law and policy.* Boston: Little, Brown, 1988.
Arbuckle JG, et al. *Environmental law handbook.* Rockville, MD: Government Institutes, 1989.
Findley RW, Farber DA. *Environmental law.* St. Paul: West, 1988.

43

Clinical Environmental Medicine

OBJECTIVES

- Discuss the relationship between epidemiology, toxicology, and the practice of environmental medicine
- Explain approaches used in the evaluation of the patient with suspected environmentally related disease

OUTLINE

KEY POINTS

- Environmental medicine can be considered to be "the study of effects upon human beings of external physical, chemical, and biologic factors in the general environment (Ducatman, 1990)." The discipline of environmental medicine "combines clinical, epidemiologic, and toxicologic approaches. It uniquely seeks to understand causation and then to adopt policy, engineering, or human factor interventions to prevent or mitigate the caused outcomes" (Ducatman, 1990).

- We can prevent environmental disease far more effectively and still more cost-effectively than we can treat it.
- Assignment of clinical or laboratory findings to environmental causes necessitates repeatability of those findings and clear epidemiologic linkage. Accuracy of diagnostic testing, in relation to exposures and efficacy of therapeutic intervention, needs to be tested by recognizable scientific means.
- The physician who practices environmental medicine is likely to encounter patients who have a variety of concerns about the potential health implications of exposure to environmental hazards. Patients rely on their physician to provide them with advice concerning sources of toxins, exposure prevention, and related public health interventions.
- In the majority of cases, the extent of the exposures are considerably less than in the traditional occupational setting.
- Clinicians who address questions about health outcomes of past or potential exposures are accorded enormous credibility. The local physician's opinion about an exposure or the cause of an outbreak is likely to be accorded more respect than the work of regulatory, public health, or research experts.
- Occupational and environmental physicians should be familiar with environmental exposure-outcome data, including their availability, methods, quality, and potential weaknesses.
- It is the responsibility of such a clinician to present exposure-outcome information in the same manner as clinical information.
- Situations that typically concern a community may involve treatment, education, and decision-making information. Such practitioners are involved directly in episodic or periodic health evaluations, diagnosis and treatment, patient and community education, implementation of public health protection, planned abatement of source stressors, exposure and outcome assessments, and disaster preparedness.

QUESTIONS

1. The focus of environmental medicine is

A. absence of usual clinical symptoms following exposures.
B. industrial hygiene control.
C. low-dose toxicology.
D. prevention.
E. significant cost savings in health care.

*2. Significant environmental exposure include all of the following **except:***

A. asbestos exposure.
B. asthma.
C. contaminated water.
D. lead exposure.
E. vinyl chloride monomer exposure.

*3. Pediatric lead poisoning concerns occur with all of the following **except:***

A. blood lead levels about 10 µg/100 ml.
B. inappropriately constructed cookware.
C. exterior latex paint.
D. older metal plumbing.
E. school-age children.

*4. All of the following tests have been used for assessing exposure to environmental hazards **except:***

A. fingernail analysis for metal poisoning.
B. measurements of cholinesterase levels for pesticide exposure.
C. hair analysis for metal exposure.
D. lead measurements in blood years after exposure.
E. x-ray fluorescence of long bones for chronic lead exposure.

REFERENCES

Agency for Toxic Substances and Disease Registry. *Case studies in environmental medicine: lead toxicity.* Washington, DC: U.S. Department of Health and Human Services, 1990.

Centers for Disease Control. *Preventing lead poisoning in young children.* Washington, DC: U.S. Department of Health and Human Services, 1991.

Ducatman AM, Chase KH, Farid I, et al. What is environmental medicine? *J. Occup Med* 32:1130, 1990.

Olin BR, et al., eds. *Facts and comparisons drug information.* St. Louis: Lippincott, December 1992 (updated monthly).

Weitzman M, et al. Lead contaminated soil abatement and urban children's blood lead levels. *J.A.M.A.* 269:1641, 1993.

44

Indoor Air Pollution

OBJECTIVES

- Discuss the relationship between indoor air pollution and health effects
- List sources that contribute to indoor air pollution
- Identify categories of pollutants that may cause indoor air pollution
- Distinguish between building-associated illness and the sick-building syndrome
- Explain various causes of chronic building-related disease
- List steps involved in the evaluation of problem buildings

OUTLINE

    I. Historical Perspective
   II. The Indoor Environment
      A. Sources of IAP
         1. External Sources
         2. Building Fabric and Interior Furnishings
         3. Mechanical Systems
         4. Occupant Generated Pollution
      B. Characterizing Indoor Air
           Table 44–1. Common sources and types of indoor contaminants
         1. Biologic Aerosols
         2. Combustion Products
         3. Particulates
         4. Pesticides
         5. Radon
         6. Volatile Organic Compounds
         7. Physical Factors
         8. The Problem Building
      C. Health Effects of IAP: Acute Building-Related Illnesses
         1. Hypersensitivity Diseases
         2. Infectious Diseases
         3. Acute and Subacute Intoxications

III. Chronic Building-Related Diseases
    A. Cancer
        1. Radon
        2. ETS and Combustion Products
        3. Particulates
        4. Volatile Organic Chemicals and Pesticides
        5. Electromagnetic Fields
    B. Neurobehavioral Disorders
    C. Pulmonary Disorders
IV. Sick-Building Syndrome
V. Mass Psychogenic Illness
VI. Multiple Chemical Sensitivities
VII. Clinical Evaluation of Building-Associated Illness
VIII. Evaluation of Problem Buildings
IX. Improving IAQ
    A. Secondary Prevention
    B. Primary Prevention
X. Conclusion
XI. References

KEY POINTS

- Indoor air pollution (IAP) is a significant and expensive health concern.
- Poor indoor air quality is not simply a matter of comfort, but may be associated with illness and death. Many toxins are present at higher levels indoors than outdoors. Lifestyle changes have led the average citizen in the United States to spend 90% of his/her life indoors. The most vulnerable segments of the population (the infirm, very young, or very old) are the most exposed.
- There are four general sources of IAP: (1) the external environment, (2) building fabric and furnishings, (3) mechanical systems, and (4) occupant-generated pollution.
- The key factors involved in indoor air quality include (1) biologic agents, (2) combustion products, (3) particulates, (4) pesticides, (5) radon, (6) volatile organic chemicals, and (7) physical factors.
- A "problem" building is one in which either more than 20% of the occupants have building-related health complaints or specific environmental contaminants have been linked with building-related illnesses. A "crisis" building is one in which complaints and public concern has reached a point where normal activities have been disrupted.
- A building-related illness is a disease with a defined pathophysiology attributable to a specific building contaminant.
- The sick-building syndrome refers to a group of transient nonspecific symptoms, affected by entering and leaving a particular building. The cause may be speculative and multifactorial.
- Indoor air pollutants have the potential for causing chronic diseases. Those of chief concern include cancer, neurobehavioral syndromes, and pulmonary disorders.
- The clinical evaluation of building-associated symptoms begins with an interview aimed at recognizing symptoms and the temporal sequence in relationship to specific environments and/or activities. Complaints of other building occupants may be relevant.
- The evaluation of a problem building should be staged. The first step involves the collection of information about the building and the complaints of occupants. Subsequently, specific environmental or medical hypotheses should be generated. "Shotgun" attempts to measure every possible pollutant should be avoided. Timing of industrial hygiene measurements may be critical.

QUESTIONS

*1. All of the following are true **except:***

A. Americans typically spend 90% of their lives indoors.
B. indoor air problems are a top priority of the EPA.
C. indoor levels of pollutants of concern rarely exceed outdoor levels.
D. poor indoor air has been associated with illness and death.
E. those most vulnerable to indoor air pollutants are often those most exposed.

*2. Each of the following contributes to workplace indoor air quality problems **except:***

A. fabrics.
B. mechanical systems.
C. occupants.
D. outdoor air.
E. drinking water purification systems.

3. The most important source of indoor radon is

A. building products.
B. cigarettes.
C. natural gas.
D. soil.
E. tap water.

4. Complaints about indoor air pollutants decrease with

A. increased weight of floor dust.
B. increased use of fleecy materials.
C. increased density on shelves.
D. decreased density of office equipment.
E. decreased ventilation.

5. Poisoning related to indoor home air pollution is most often related to:

A. asbestos.
B. carbon monoxide.
C. cleaning products.
D. pesticides.
E. radon.

REFERENCE

Menzies R, et al. The effect of varying levels of outdoor air supply in the symptom of sick building syndrome. *N. Engl. J. Med.* 328:821, 1993.

45

The Agency for Toxic Substances

OBJECTIVES

- State the mission of ATSDR
- Explain the difference between a public health assessment and consultation from ATSDR
- List the educational objectives of this agency

OUTLINE

KEY POINTS

- The Superfund legislation created the Agency for Toxic Substances and Disease Registry (ATSDR) to help in understanding the human health impact of environmental chemical contamination. The agency's mission is "to prevent or mitigate adverse effects to both human health and the quality of life resulting from exposure to hazardous substances in the environment."

- A public health assessment may be conducted by this agency to evaluate "data and information on the release of hazardous substances into the environment to assess any current or future impact on public health."
- The agency may also provide health consultation, a less inclusive response to a request for information about health risks from a specific site.
- When performing a public health assessment, the agency makes efforts to include information about the community health concerns in their report.
- ATSDR is available for consultation by physicians working with environmentally related situations.
- ATSDR has developed and is producing informational publications aimed specifically at environmental situations. These include *Toxicological Profiles,* which are monographs on the health effects of specific hazardous substances, and *Case Studies in Environmental Medicine,* which are self-instructional exercises.

QUESTIONS

1. In terms of hazardous waste

A. approximately 50 million tons are produced yearly.
B. there are approximately 100,000 documented hazardous waste sites.
C. the estimated cost of site clean-up is $5 billion.
D. national priority sites number about 1,300.
E. toxic wastes are found only at factory and former factory sites.

2. The most important aspect of assessing the likelihood of environmental disease is

A. the evaluation of environmental data.
B. the complete medical history.
C. the laboratory examination.
D. the physical examination.
E. the reference to occupational regulations.

3. Primary treatment for many environmentally related conditions is

A. detoxification.
B. pharmacological agents.
C. psychological referral.
D. reassurance.
E. removal from exposure.

*4. Which of the following is **false** regarding the ATSDR?*

A. ATSDR has specifically been designated with regulatory and enforcement powers by the Superfund.
B. ATSDR develops educational materials primarily in the form of case studies.
C. ATSDR's relationship to EPA parallels NIOSH's relationship to OSHA.
D. Superfund legislation created the ATSDR.
E. ATSDR's primary mission is to prevent or mitigate adverse health effects from the environment.

REFERENCE

U.S. Government Printing Office. *Federal Register* 54:33617, August 15, 1989.

46

Environmental Medical Emergencies

OBJECTIVES

- List components of the work-site emergency response which are relevant to physicians
- Explain OSHA requirements for emergency responders

OUTLINE

    I. First Aid and Emergency Medical Care
   II. Protection of Emergency Response Personnel
 III. Provision of Emergency Medical Information
 IV. Medical Surveillance
   V. Coordination with Community Health Care Providers

KEY POINTS

- Occupational physicians are likely to be involved in the development and implementation of work-site emergency response plans.
- Work-site emergency response requirements of relevance may include (1) first aid and emergency medical care, (2) protection of emergency response personnel, (3) provision of emergency medical information, (4) medical surveillance, and (5) coordination with community health care providers.
- OSHA and EPA require that an emergency response plan be developed and implemented before the start of hazardous waste and emergency response operations at a facility.
- Employers must assure that response personnel are physically able to use the provided equipment. This requires the professional involvement of a physician and updated medical information.

- Work sites at which hazardous substances are processed or stored should have detailed medical information available on the specific health effects of exposure to those substances.
- Employers are required to develop medical surveillance programs for emergency response personnel and other employees involved in hazardous materials emergencies.
- Important components of a facility's emergency response plans are explicit agreements between the facility and surrounding community emergency response organizations, including EMS providers and hospitals.

QUESTIONS

1. Work-site emergency preparedness for environmental disasters requires each of the following **except:**

A. coordination with community health units.
B. first-aid services.
C. medical surveillance.
D. mobile testing lab or labs.
E. the provision of emergency medical information.

2. A workplace medical surveillance program for emergency response personnel

A. attempts to find all sick individuals.
B. is defined by NIOSH.
C. is mandated by OSHA and EPA.
D. is at the employer's discretion.
E. is prohibited by ADA.

3. Emergency response plans should include coordination with

A. EMS organizations.
B. fire departments.
C. hospitals.
D. police departments.
E. all of the above.

4. Protection of emergency response personnel must include all of the above **except:**

A. determination of physical ability to use a respirator.
B. availability of hepatitis B vaccination.
C. provision of a self-contained breathing apparatus (SCBA).
D. annual chest x-rays and pulmonary function testing.
E. procedures for monitoring vital signs when using impermeable suits and heavy equipment.

47

Emergency Response to Environmental Incidents

OBJECTIVES

- Identify sources of assistance in chemical emergencies
- List the components of a risk inventory from a facility survey
- Explain factors that determine the level of appropriate emergency response
- Discuss importance of debriefing after an emergency response plan is activated

OUTLINE

     G. Decontamination
     H. Containment of Incident
     I. Evacuation and Site Security
     J. Systems of Outside Notification
     K. Site Communications
     L. Role of Outside Agencies
     M. Public Relations
     N. Debriefing
  III. Role of the Occupational Physician
  IV. Summary
   V. References

KEY POINTS

- The emergency response to environmental incidents combines the principles of occupational medicine and emergency medicine.
- Unexpected events that challenge routine capabilities of local and regional emergency response systems are known as mass casualty incidents.
- The potential for mishaps with hazardous materials is underscored by the fact that approximately 4 billion tons of regulated materials are transported annually in the United States.
- The Chemical Transportation Emergency Center (CHEMTREC), a service of the Chemical Manufacturer's Association that provides assistance in transportation incidents, received over 48,000 calls related to hazardous materials (HAZMAT) emergencies from 1986 through 1991.
- To properly advise the planning for hazardous material emergencies, the physician must have a firm understanding of the toxicity of chemicals used at various sites. By conducting a facility survey of materials used and their respective processes, a risk inventory can be developed.
- To deal effectively with unexpected releases of hazardous materials, an emergency response plan (ERP) should consider the following: (1) exposures may affect a single worker or result in a mass casualty incident, (2) necessary contacts and information sources need to be outlined, and (3) guidelines should be prepared for grading the response.
- The response plan should address issues such as (1) the types of events that will trigger the ERP, and the corresponding level of response; (2) the responsibilities of the response team; (3) the relationship with neighboring businesses; and (4) the role and contact mechanisms for government agencies.
- Selection of personal protective equipment or chemical protective clothing requires knowledge of substances to which the garment will be exposed, and the duration of such exposure.
- The level of response appropriate for a given incident should be determined by the level of technical expertise necessary to control the material(s), the presence of fire or explosion hazards, and the potential radius of risk.
- To prevent confusion, a clear chain of command is critical in the event of an incident.
- Decontamination issues must also be included in the response plan.
- After activation of the ERP, debriefings are important, with evaluation of events leading up to the incident, and attention to prevention of similar events.

QUESTIONS

*1. All of the following are regulated when shipped under Department of Transportation (DOT) standards **except:***

A. benzene.

B. canola oil.
C. milk.
D. sulfuric acid.
E. trichloroethane.

2. *As part of decontamination procedures associated with environmental spills, which of the following is **least** necessary?*

A. Changes of clothing
B. Disposal equipment for suits
C. First-aid services
D. Shower facilities
E. Respiratory protection

3. *Hazardous materials evacuation plans*

A. should be part of right-to-know orientation.
B. should be filed with local government agencies.
C. must have contingencies for weather, explosions, and fires.
D. require a command center.
E. all of the above.

4. *For emergency response activities, notification checklists for outside callers should include all of the following **except:***

A. location of incident.
B. material involved.
C. underlying cause of accident.
D. age of victims.
E. extent of injuries or symptoms.

5. *When an environmental emergency occurs the public relations plan should focus on:*

A. EMS response.
B. local funeral home directors.
C. local media.
D. regulatory agencies with oversight.
E. shareholders, if a public corporation.

REFERENCE

Code of Federal Regulations, Title 49, part 172, section 101 (commonly referred to as 49 CFR 171.101).

48

Accessing Environmental Data

OBJECTIVES

- Discuss the types and sources of data that may help with diagnosis and management of suspected environmental health problems
- Explain the assessment of the quality of data

OUTLINE

KEY POINTS

- A variety of environmental data collection systems exist in the United States. Some exist because of regulatory requirements.
- For a true picture of human exposure to emerge, the practitioner must address the cumulative nature of exposure from multiple pathways, including exposure by der-

mal and respiratory routes, as well as by ingestion. The magnitude, duration, and frequency of exposure must also be considered.
- Two on-line data systems that may provide the practitioner with general information regarding an agent are the Toxicology Information (TOXLINE) and Toxicology Data Network (TOXNET).
- Many federal and state agencies are responsible for the collection and dissemination of environmental data. Some of these include the Agency for Toxic Substances and Disease Registry (ATSDR), the Environmental Protection Agency (EPA), and various state departments.

QUESTIONS

*1. Which of the following factors is **least** important in population assessment?*

A. Duration of exposure
B. Food chain exposures
C. Frequency of exposure
D. Magnitude of exposure
E. Single pathway exposure assessment

2. Computer accessible databases include:

A. Medline.
B. Medlars.
C. Grateful Med.
D. Toxline.
E. all of the above.

3. NIOSH maintains

A. Toxnet.
B. Medlars.
C. Medline.
D. RTECS.
E. Zipline.

*4. All of the following are responsible for collection and dissemination of environmental data **except:***

A. ATSDR.
B. EPA.
C. OSHA.
D. State health departments.
E. Department of Agriculture.

49

The Environmental Audit

OBJECTIVES

- Identify the objectives of an environmental audit
- Discuss the role of the occupational and environmental medicine physician in an audit team

OUTLINE

    I. The Role of the Environmental Audit
   II. The Timing of the Environmental Audit
  III. The Legal Basis
  IV. Conducting the Audit
   V. The Role of the Occupational and Environmental Physician
  VI. References

KEY POINTS

- An environmental audit is a process that includes the gathering of information on activities at a facility that may impact the environment or human health, especially any activities subject to legal or regulatory requirements.
- The most important role of the environmental audit is to ensure regulatory compliance, and prevent violations, fines, public relations problems, and even criminal charges.
- An environmental audit may be appropriate on a regularly scheduled basis, at the time of changing or upgrading facilities, during divestiture or acquisition, and in anticipation of an external audit.
- The first step in an environmental audit is information gathering. Later a site visit will focus on the entire process from raw materials to final product. At the conclusion of the site visit, an exit interview is usually held. A staged follow-up action plan may also be included.

QUESTIONS

1. The most important role of the environmental audit is

A. anticipate regulatory reform.
B. increase insurance coverage.
C. information for occupational physicians.
D. regulatory compliance.
E. toxic tort reform.

2. It is appropriate to conduct environmental audits in each of the following time frames:

A. at time of plant upgrade.
B. divestiture of properties.
C. on a 1- to 3-year cycle.
D. prior to external audit.
E. all of the above.

*3. Each of the following is an appropriate role for the environmental physician in regards to audits **except:***

A. to assist in report writing.
B. to direct laboratory testing.
C. to interpret results for management.
D. to review audit results.
E. to serve as a team member.

50

Environmental Risk Assessment

OBJECTIVES

- Explain the usefulness of risk assessment
- List types of information used in the formation of a risk assessment
- Distinguish between NOAEL and LOAEL
- Recognize levels in the IARC cancer classification system

OUTLINE

I. The Risk Assessment Process
    Figure 50–1. NAS/NRC risk assessment/management paradigm
II. Approaches to Acquiring Information
III. Approaches to Conducting Risk Assessment
    A. Noncancer Endpoints
        Table 50–1. Use of uncertainty factors in deriving reference dose
    B. Cancer
        Table 50–2. IARC cancer classification
        Table 50–3. EPA and IARC carcinogenicity groupings
IV. The Occupational and Environmental Physician
V. References

KEY POINTS

- Low-level exposures that may produce chronic diseases, particularly neoplasms, are often managed through the process of qualitative or quantitative risk assessment. These assessments are also used for policy decisions at local, state, and federal levels, and in multiple regulatory settings.
- Qualitative risk assessment is commonly performed by "authoritative bodies" including the International Agency for Research on Cancer (IARC), the American Conference of Governmental Industry Hygienists (ACGIH), the Environmental Protection Agency (EPA), and others.

- The risk assessment process involves four steps: (1) hazard identification, (2) exposure-dose-response relationship, (3) exposure assessment, and (4) risk characterization.
- Clinical and epidemiologic studies are especially useful in that data are obtained on people. Laboratory animal studies, like controlled human exposure studies, have the advantage of using carefully defined conditions matched to experimental needs. In vitro studies that use cells and tissues from people and laboratory animals represent the ultimate "reductionist" approach of defining pollutant effects.
- The approach used by the ACGIH and the EPA for noncancer end points makes use of safety or uncertainty factors to extrapolate from levels of observed effect or absence of effect to levels of exposure that may be viewed as acceptable.
- LOAEL = lowest observed adverse effect level; NOAEL = no observable effect level.
- The IARC conducts a formalized risk assessment that leads to a qualitative clarification of a compound's carcinogenic potential. The evaluation process considers three types of data: human carcinogenicity data, experimental carcinogenicity data, and supporting evidence of carcinogenicity. The evidence of carcinogenicity is classified into four categories: Group 1 includes chemicals and processes established as human carcinogens. Group 2 includes those that are probably (Group 2A) or possibly (Group 2B) carcinogenic to humans. Group 3 includes agents that are not classified. Group 4 includes agents that are probably not carcinogenic.

QUESTIONS

1. *Each of the following organizations conducts carcinogen assessment studies* ***except:***

A. American Conference of Governmental Industrial Hygienists (ACGIH).
B. Consumer Product Safety Commission (CPSC).
C. Environmental Protection Agency (EPA).
D. International Agency for Research on Cancer (IARC).
E. National Toxicology Program (NTP).

2. *The risk assessment process includes each of the following* ***except:***

A. exposure assessment.
B. exposure dose-response assessment.
C. hazard identification.
D. personal exposure measurement.
E. risk characterization.

3. *Risk assessment is best approached with*

A. clinical data on individual patients.
B. computer models.
C. epidemiologic data.
D. laboratory animal studies.
E. laboratory based human exposures.

4. *When assessing the carcinogenic potential of a compound, the most relevant information for regulatory purposes is*

A. animal data.
B. chemical composition.
C. human data.

D. mechanistic data.

E. threshold level.

5. *Which of the following risk assessment data are useful to the environmental physician?*

A. Communication of risk

B. Disease potential in work force

C. Plausibility of association

D. Risk identification

E. All of the above

REFERENCE

National Academy of Sciences/National Research Council. *Risk assessment in the federal government: managing the process.* Washington, DC: National Academy Press, 1983.

Section 5 Answers

CHAPTER 41 ANSWERS

1. The answer is D. (Reference: p. 606)

Global warming is likely to produce exaggerations in existing weather trends and make extreme weather conditions more frequent.

2. The answer is D. (Reference: p. 608)

The human health effects of increased ultraviolet irradiation due to ozone depletion include higher risks of nonmelanoma skin cancer (particularly squamous cell carcinoma and actinic keratitis, a premalignant condition), malignant melanoma (Charman, 1990; Henriksen et al., 1990; Kripke, 1990; Longstreth, 1988; Morison, 1989; Olson, 1989; van Kuijk, 1991; Vitasa et al., 1990), cataract and retinal degeneration, and possibly impaired immunologic responses (Morison, 1989).

3. The answer is B. (Reference: p. 609)

Our recent population growth is not the first population explosion humankind has experienced. In fact, this process has occurred at least twice before. The first population explosion occurred about 100,000 B.C., when our ancestors learned how to organize into tribes, make stone tools, and hunt larger animals. The second surge appears to have occurred about 5,000 B.C., when humankind developed agriculture. In both of these prehistoric events, the big change came in the ability to produce food. With the coming of the Industrial Revolution, two changes occurred. Industry and more efficient agriculture allowed humankind to support a larger population. At the same time, improved public health and medical care both prolonged the average life span and increased the number of individuals who survived to bear children.

4. The answer is D. (Reference: p. 610)

Agricultural production has expanded enormously since then; essentially all the arable land in most parts of the world is under cultivation. The world has adopted the strategy of increasing the yield per acre by heavy fertilization and development of new crop strains. Even with the rapid spread of this Green Revolution, however, world food production has been increasing only at about 4.5% per year overall and has actually been falling in Africa. By comparison, the world population is increasing by about 1.6% per year, which leaves a bare margin for improvement of chronic malnutrition in the underdeveloped world. This progress can be reversed at any time. In 1972, for example, the monsoons erased most of the progress India had made. In 1973, the United States lost over 40% of its corn crop in the South to a fungus because the new high-yield strain was exceptionally susceptible. In the 1980s, overgrazing and overpopulation led to a terrible famine in sub-Saharan Africa. The Green Revolution is fragile and easily thwarted because it is expensive, requires education, depends on ideal weather, and puts farm laborers out of work in countries where there are no other jobs (The environment and population growth: decade for action, 1992).

5. The answer is C. (Reference: pp. 610, 611)

Sustainable development is a concept critical to understanding solutions to large-scale ecologic degradation and resource depletion. Sustainable development involves establishing an economic structure that ideally consumes only as much as the natural environment produces and emits only as much as the natural environment can absorb.

CHAPTER 42 ANSWERS

1. The answer is B. (Reference: p. 614)

The primary prevention of environmental exposure and disease is implemented by the combination of local, state, and federal regulations. In contrast to human risk-based occupational standards, many environmental regulations are oriented to minimize exposure by controlling emissions of categories of pollutants according to medium of exposure. However, environmental regulations are being carefully scrutinized to determine their impact on human health risk, an area of expertise for occupational and environmental physicians.

To comprehend the current approach to the prevention of environmental disease, one must understand the regulatory framework as well as the science that supports these rules. These prevention-based regulations serve as the basis for the control of hazardous exposure and, ultimately, prevention of disease. In fact, exposure control strategies must be recommended with clear knowledge of applicable regulations.

2. The answer is B. (Reference: p. 614)

Environmental regulations mirror public concern and its reflection of actual risk. As a result, regulations in the United States and other countries have been driven by a series of environmental issues, many of which arose from catastrophic situations. The EPA was established in 1970 by Congress one year after a major oil spill off the coast of California. The formation of the EPA unified federal regulation of the environment under one federal agency. The EPA's charter included all media: air, water, and solid and hazardous waste (including liquid waste). The EPA began a sequential review and tightening of federal environmental protection regulation in the early 1970s (Anderson and Mandelker, 1988; Arbuckle et al., 1989; Findley and Farber, 1988).

3. The answer is A. (Reference: p. 615)

In 1986, CERCLA amendments, including another extension of the scope of environmental oversight with EPCRA, were passed. In the aftermath of Bhopal, EPCRA requires industries to notify governmental authorities of the hazardous substances located on a site.

4. The answer is B. (Reference: p. 617)

Exceedences and unusual emissions must be reported under CAA and Emergency Right to Know provisions. These publicly available reports can provide excellent exposure data in evaluating an individual case or cluster of cases.

5. The answer is D. (Reference: p. 617)

The CWA has the following five major components: (1) a system of minimum national effluent guidelines, (2) water quality standards, (3) discharge permit programs, (4) provisions for special issues such as toxics, and (5) a grant program for publicly owned treatment works (POTWs).

Storm water runoff is also regulated by the CWA.

Failures to meet discharge requirements for effluent or storm water must be reported to the EPA, normally at the state level.

Significant storage tank regulations also exist (under RCRA).

CHAPTER 43 ANSWERS

1. The answer is D. (Reference: p. 623)

Environmental medicine can be considered to be the study of effects upon human beings of external physical, chemical, and biologic factors in the general environment.

2. The answer is E. (Reference: Table 43–1)

3. The answer is A. (Reference: pp. 625, 626)

Office referrals generally begin when childhood lead levels exceed 10 g/100 ml of whole blood. This referral level from the Centers for Disease Control recommendations is based on a strong and steadily growing body of evidence that low-level lead intoxication causes significant intellect deficit in the developing fetus and young child (Agency for Toxic Substances and Disease Registry, 1990; Centers for Disease Control, 1991; Olin et al., 1992; Ruff, 1993; Weitzman, 1993).

4. The answer is D. (Reference: p. 629)

For some exposures, biologic monitoring can be used to augment assessments of past exposures. Substances with long body half-lives are most accessible to biologic monitoring, particularly when partitioning is in equilibration with accessible body tissues (e.g., blood, urine, hair, and nails). Concerns about lead exposure can be addressed in individuals or in populations routinely. The routine schedule for biologic monitoring of environmental lead in children is blood level measured at ages 1 and 2 for low-risk children, more frequently for children at high risk (Agency for Toxic Substances and Disease Registry, 1990; Centers for Disease Control, 1991) (Table 43–5). With slightly more effort, other heavy metals or polycyclic halogenated hydrocarbon exposures can be measured. These determinations provide valuable population and individual information in the event that the levels are elevated.

Table 43–1. *Examples of office encounters in environmental medicine[a]*

Issue	Population
Lead exposure	Children, home renovators, hobbyists
Building-related complaints	Schoolchildren and their parents, home renovators, and tenants
Puzzling symptoms attributed to chemicals	See Multiple Chemical Sensitivity
Environmental cancer concerns	Residents near power lines, abandoned older (asbestos-containing) buildings, waste or incineration sites, areas with radon problems; residents with contaminated water
Reproductive concerns	See also Lead, Hobbies, Environmental Cancer
Pulmonary disease (asthma, colds, bronchitis)	Residents near power plants or industries

[a]As in the rest of medicine, causation is a decision, not a certain implication of any encounter.

CHAPTER 44 ANSWERS

1. The answer is C. (Reference: p. 633)

As research progressed through the late 1980s, the federal government recognized IAP as a significant and expensive health concern. Investigators found that:
Poor indoor air quality (IAQ) was not simply a matter of comfort, but was associated with illness and death.
Many toxins were present at higher levels indoors than outdoors.
Changes in lifestyle over the last century had led average citizens of the United States to spend 90% of their lives indoors.
The most vulnerable segments of our population, the infirm, the very young, and the very old, were the most exposed.
These revelations led the EPA to place IAP among the top environmental priorities.

2. The answer is E. (Reference: p. 634)

Four sources contribute to IAP: external environment, building fabric, mechanical systems, and occupants.

3. The answer is D. (Reference: p. 637)

The bulk of radon enters buildings as a soil gas, though other sources include tap water from private wells, building products, and, minimally, natural gas. As a soil gas, radon primarily affects the lower levels of a building; concentrations of radon tend to decrease in higher levels.

4. The answer is D. (Reference: p. 638)

Users of photocopiers, carbonless copy paper, and video display terminals were more likely to have building-related complaints. Complaint rates are more closely related to the intensity of pollution sources than to ventilation rates (Menzies et al., 1993).

5. The answer is B. (Reference: p. 640)

Though carbon monoxide poisoning rarely occurs in office settings, it is a leading cause of poisoning at home. About 1,800 accidental deaths occur annually.

CHAPTER 45 ANSWERS

1. The answer is D. (Reference: p. 651)

The Environmental Protection Agency (EPA) currently includes 33,000 sites in its inventory of known hazardous waste sites. Of that number, about 1,270 are on the National Priority List (NPL), which is a group of sites that the EPA considers its highest priority for remediation. The EPA has estimated that cleaning up the current NPL sites may cost more than $30 billion.

2. The answer is B. (Reference: p. 655)

The history is the fundamental tool for any environmental investigation, and it must include all of the patient's environments, occupational and otherwise.

3. The answer is E. (Reference: p. 656)

Central to the treatment of environmentally related illnesses usually is removal of patients from the source of the contaminants affecting them. While other, more traditional, medical care may be useful, the primary goal should be the elimination of pathways between the patient and the environmental contaminant.

4. The answer is A. (Reference: p. 652, Table 45–1)

Although the Superfund Act is administered principally by the EPA, a new agency, the ATSDR, was formed to help in understanding the human health impact of widespread environmental chemical contamination. The Superfund legislation created this agency to consider the harmful health effects that may be associated with hazardous waste.

The relationship between the EPA and ATSDR is, in some ways, similar to that of the Occupational Safety and Health Administration (OSHA) and the National Institute for Occupational Safety and Health (NIOSH), in that the regulatory and enforcement powers reside with the EPA. ATSDR's mission is to prevent or mitigate adverse effects to both human health and the quality of life resulting from exposure to hazardous substances in the environment (U.S. Government Printing Office, 1989).

Table 45–1. *Legislative mandates and the Agency for Toxic Substances and Disease Registry (ATSDR) response*

Legislative mandate	ATSDR response
Overall public health implications of a hazardous waste site	Public health assessment
Specific questions concerning a site	Health consultation
Toxicologic information of site contaminants	Toxicologic profile
Health surveillance of affected residents	Epidemiologic studies and registries
Educational and training materials	Case studies in environmental medicine, courses for physicians
Applied and substance-specific research	Sponsorship of intramural and academic research programs, conferences, etc.
Response to emergencies involving hazardous substances	24-hour emergency response capability including on site, if required

CHAPTER 46 ANSWERS

1. The answer is D. (Reference: p. 660)

Work-site emergency response requirements of relevance to occupational physicians are grouped and discussed according to the following five types of response functions and activities:

1. First aid and emergency medical care
2. Protection of emergency response personnel
3. Provision of emergency medical information
4. Medical surveillance
5. Coordination with community health care providers.

2. The answer is C. (Reference: p. 663)

OSHA (29 CFR 1910.120) and the EPA (40 CFR 311) require employers to develop medical surveillance programs for emergency response personnel and other employees involved in hazardous materials emergencies.

3. The answer is E. (Reference: p. 663)

Important components of facility emergency response plans are explicit agreements between the facility and the surrounding community's emergency response organizations, including EMS organizations and hospitals.

4. The answer is D. (Reference: p. 661)

Emergency response personnel are exposed to greater variety and severity of health risks than are most other employees. For example, fire fighters regularly risk thermal injuries, toxic exposures, and trauma. Likewise, emergency medical technicians (EMT) and emergency physicians are at greater risk of blood-borne diseases than are most other health care workers. Employers are obliged by OSHA (and, in some cases, by the EPA) to provide acceptable levels of protection to those personnel. The occupational physician plays an important role in assuring that adequate protection is actually available to response personnel.

Use of respirators is one example. OSHA requires that SCBA be provided to and used by members of industrial fire brigades (29 CFR 1910.156) and emergency personnel responding to hazardous materials releases (29 CFR 1910.120).

CHAPTER 47 ANSWERS

1. The answer is C. (Reference: p. 667)

To regulate interstate transportation, the Department of Transportation (DOT) uses nine major classifications of regulated materials, including nearly 3,000 individual substances (Code of Federal Regulations, Title 49, part 172, Section 101) (Table 47–3). The final DOT category, "other regulated materials," contains many seemingly innocuous substances that represent hazards on the ecosystem level.

2. The answer is E. (Reference: p. 675)

It is often best to set up the decontamination zone in a corridor with progressive stations that move from fully contaminated to fully clean. Possible stations could include:

Initial shower/cleansing of exterior of PPE
Removal of PPE
Removal of any undergarments that may have been contaminated with leakage of the outer PPE
Personal shower/cleansing
Medical station for any immediate monitoring needs

3. The answer is E. (Reference: p. 676)

Like fire escape plans, hazardous materials evacuation plans should be established. Plans should be posted and reviewed as part of the right to know (RTK) orientation. Regional evacuation plans should be filed with the local government agency responsible for coordinating the responses of other services.

Plans for community evacuations must have contingencies for weather, explosions, and fires. Computers linked through modems to the National Weather Service for local and regional monitoring can assist in predicting evacuation needs. Computer programs are available that aid a sophisticated command center to make predictions regarding dispersion of any particular substance in light of local climate conditions.

4. The answer is D. (Reference: p. 676)

Emergency notification procedures should include a checklist of information to be provided at the time of contacting respondents. This checklist should be prominently posted next to each telephone that might be used for notification and include the following:

Telephone number from which the call is coming
Name and location of the caller and facility/site
Time and location of the incident
Nature of incident (e.g., spill, explosion, confined space)
Material involved
Number of victims and extent of injuries
Condition and/or signs and symptoms of the victims
Name and phone number of safety officer responsible for the area of operations involved in the incident

5. The answer is C. (Reference: p. 677)

A plan to notify and cooperate with local media to disseminate necessary information is essential.

CHAPTER 48 ANSWERS

1. The answer is E. (Reference: p. 684)

For a true picture of human exposure to emerge, the practitioner must address the cumulative nature of exposure from multiple pathways, including routes of exposure such as dermal, respiratory, and ingestion. Any such consideration must include the impact of food chain exposures, especially for substances readily stored (lead) or concentrated selectively in certain tissues, such as polychlorinated biphenyls (PCBs) in fat. Other factors to consider in relation to a patient's health include:

Magnitude of exposure: What is the effective concentration in biologic media? Measures of magnitude will be more likely expressed in a volume of environmental media such as air or water.

Duration of exposure: How long was the actual exposure? Acute or chronic exposure? A particular concern is whether sharp spikes in concentration for short periods may be relevant.

Frequency of exposure: How often does this exposure occur? Does it vary seasonally or temporally?

2. The answer is E. (Reference: p. 684)

Agent-specific information concerning the toxicologic characteristics may be of use to practitioners in assessing the potential for health effects in a specific case. Two on-line data systems that can provide the practitioner with general information regarding an agent are the Toxicology Information (TOXLINE) and Toxicology Data Network (TOXNET). Both are supported by the MEDLARS management section of the National Library of Medicine. TOXLINE is composed of 16 subfiles, and TOXNET of 10 files, many of which could be of particular interest to the practitioner.

3. The answer is D. (Reference: p. 684)

The Registry of Toxic Effects of Chemical Substances (RTECS) is maintained by the National Institute for Occupational Safety and Health. This file contains information on agent-specific characteristics including toxicity in both humans and animals and other characteristics of importance to clinicians.

4. The answer is C. (Reference: pp. 685, 686)

Many federal and state agencies are responsible for the collection and dissemination of environmental data. This chapter focuses on the agencies listed here because of their singular importance to environmental health.

Agency for Toxic Substances and Disease Registry
Environmental Protection Agency
State Health and Environmental Departments

CHAPTER 49 ANSWERS

1. The answer is D. (Reference: p. 693)

The most important role of the environmental audit is to ensure regulatory compliance and prevent violations, fines, public relations problems, and even criminal charges.

2. The answer is E. (Reference: p. 694)

There are several occasions on which environmental audits should be conducted: (1) as an ongoing review of environmental programs—regular review (e.g., 1–3 years) is commonly scheduled by major industries; (2) at the time of the decision to invest in new or upgraded existing facilities; (3) during acquisition and divestitures; and (4) in anticipation of an external audit.

3. The answer is B. (Reference: pp. 695, 696)

Occupational and environmental medicine (OEM) physicians may be a part of the environmental audit team, review the audit report, or be informed users of it. The OEM physician has a unique understanding of the relationship between human health and environmental exposure. Although the audit commonly focuses on regulatory compliance, protection of human health is the ultimate goal of regulations. In fact, many regulations essentially require an assessment of health risk. As a result, the OEM physician may increasingly become a part of the audit team and participate in report preparation.

A second role for the OEM physician is to review the audit. This activity may focus on the accuracy of the observations and conclusions, especially the implications of the audit on the health of the work force or community, or both, and the need for preventive actions. Although the audit does not usually include an initial action plan, a plan is commonly generated for each major observation noted in the audit. Implementing and integrating the substance of this plan with ongoing health programs is an important activity that may require the knowledge of an OEM physician. For example, particularly in acquisition audits, the representative sampling of soils and final products will be conducted.

A third interface of the OEM physician with environmental auditing is to use the data, especially exposure sampling findings, modeling results, and risk assessment reports. This information may prove useful in evaluating a clinical case or an illness among groups of individuals, or in communicating risk to members of the community. Reliable data should be preferentially used, especially those that document exposure, concentration, biologic dose, and potential health effect.

CHAPTER 50 ANSWERS

1. The answer is B. (Reference: p. 697)

Qualitative risk assessment is commonly performed by authoritative bodies, including the International Agency for Research on Cancer (IARC), American Conference of Governmental Industry Hygienists (ACGIH), Environmental Protection Agency (EPA), National Toxicology Program (NTP), and other agencies. These organizations weigh available evidence and categorize carcinogens or safe levels for exposure to toxicants.

2. The answer is D. (Reference: p. 697)

The risk assessment process, as codified by the National Academy of Sciences (NAS), involves four steps. The first, hazard identification, is qualitative; that is, it assesses the toxicant's potential for causing health effects. The second, exposure-dose-response assessment, establishes a quantitative relationship between exposure and response. Both of these steps use human data if available. In the absence of comprehensive human data (which is usually the case), information from studies with laboratory animals, cells, and/or tissues from animals and people must be used. Exposure assessment, the third step, may use actual measurements or, more frequently, results obtained by modeling. The fourth and final step, risk characterization, involves integration of results from steps 2 and 3 to assess risk for the specific exposure scenario under consideration (Fig. 50–1) (National Academy of Sciences/National Research Council, 1983).

3. The answer is C. (Reference: p. 698)

Clinical and epidemiologic studies are especially useful in that the data are obtained on people.

4. The answer is C. (Reference: p. 701)

The evaluation process considers three types of data: human carcinogenicity data, experimental carcinogenicity data, and supporting evidence of carcinogenicity. Definitive evidence of human carcinogenicity can only be obtained from epidemiologic or clinical studies.

5. The answer is C. (Reference: pp. 704, 705)

Specific knowledge of the actual occupational and environmental exposure situation may be most important. The extent to which the agent is respirable must be considered in evaluating exposure to fibers and particles. The likelihood of a particular route of exposure actually occurring as well as the comparative level of occupational or environmental exposure is of crucial importance in determining the actual human risk.

Further, the occupational and environmental medicine (OEM) physician has a role both in standard-setting process through risk assessment and interpreting the standards based on knowledge of the specific situation. When regulations are proposed, it is not always possible to analyze each integral element of the risk assessment process. Key questions should be posed and default assumptions and risk characterizations challenged, when appropriate, by OEM physicians. Risk assessments based on regulatory guidelines always need to be considered as candidates for refinement based on specific knowledge.

In summary, risk assessment, qualitative and quantitative, can be instrumental in environmental medicine. This approach must be carefully integrated with clinical assessments. Furthermore, the clinician should take an active part in the determination of risk assessment when appropriate and in the examination of qualitative or quantitative risk assessments that are used in formulating regulatory policies or enforcement proceedings.

Subject Index